easy gluten-free

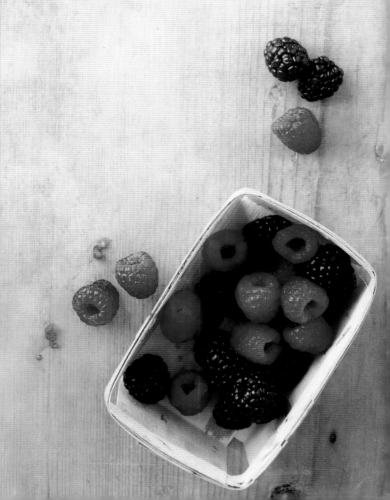

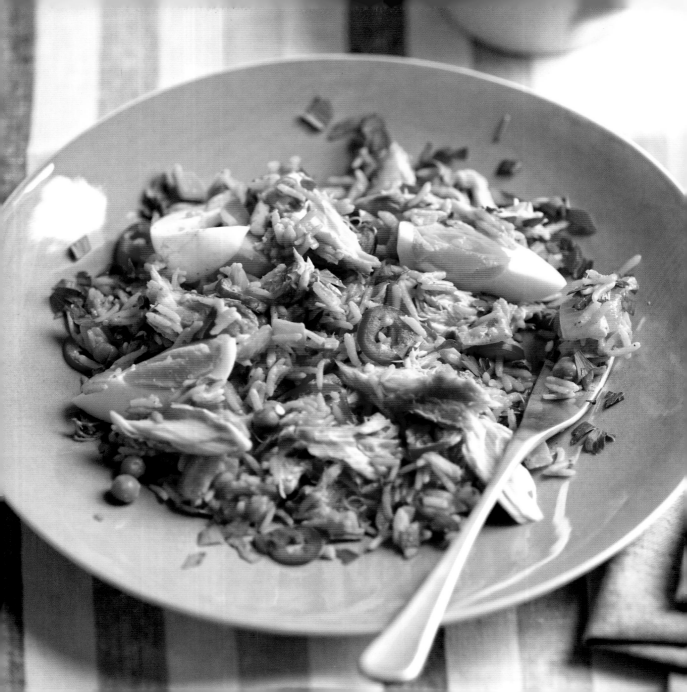

easy gluten-free

simple recipes for delicious food every day

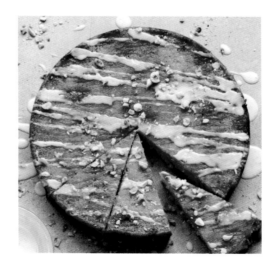

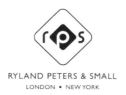

RYLAND PETERS & SMALL
LONDON • NEW YORK

Designer Paul Stradling
Editors Miriam Catley and Lesley Malkin
Production Mai-Ling Collyer
Art Director Leslie Harrington
Editorial Director Julia Charles
Publisher Cindy Richards

Indexer Vanessa Bird

Published in 2018 by
Ryland Peters & Small
20–21 Jockey's Fields
London WC1R 4BW
and
341 E 116th St
New York NY 10029

www.rylandpeters.com

Recipe collection compiled by Julia
Charles. Text © Miranda Ballard, Jessica
Bourke, Jordan Bourke, Ursula Ferrigno,
Amy Ruth Finegold, Mat Follas, Liz Franklin,
Victoria Glass, Dunja Gulin, Victoria Hall,
Carole Hilker, Jenny Linford, Hannah Miles,
Rosa Rigby, Laura Washburn, Jenna Zoe
and Ryland Peters & Small 2018

Design and photographs © Ryland Peters
& Small 2018

ISBN: 978-1-84975-940-3

10 9 8 7 6 5 4 3 2 1

A CIP record for this book is available from
the British Library.
US Library of Congress Cataloging-in-
Publication data has been applied for.

Printed and bound in China

notes

• Both British (Metric) and American (Imperial plus US cups) are included in
these recipes for your convenience; however, it is important to work with one
set of measurements and not alternate between the two within a recipe.

• All spoon measurements are level unless otherwise specified.

• All eggs are medium (UK) or large (US), unless specified as large, in which
case US extra-large should be used. Uncooked or partially cooked eggs
should not be served to the very old, frail, young children, pregnant women or
those with compromised immune systems. Eggs do not contain gluten and are
safe for use following the recipes in this book.

• Ovens should be preheated to the specified temperatures. We recommend
using an oven thermometer. If using a fan-assisted oven, adjust temperatures
according to the manufacturer's instructions.

• When a recipe calls for the grated zest of citrus fruit, buy unwaxed fruit and
wash well before using. If you can only find treated fruit, scrub well in warm
soapy water before using.

• If you believe that you may have a gluten intolerance or coeliac disease,
it is essential to seek professional medical advice. Once you have been
diagnosed with either, there are many sources of information available to you.
The Coeliac Societies in the UK and USA are able to provide a large amount
of advice and support.

• Disclaimer: The views expressed in this book are general views only
and readers are urged to consult a relevant and qualified specialist or
physician for individual advice before beginning any dietary regimen.
Ryland Peters & Small hereby exclude all liability to the extent
permitted by law for any errors or omissions in this book and
for any loss, damage or expense (whether direct or indirect)
suffered by a third party relying on any information
contained in this book.

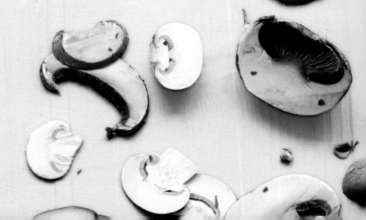

contents

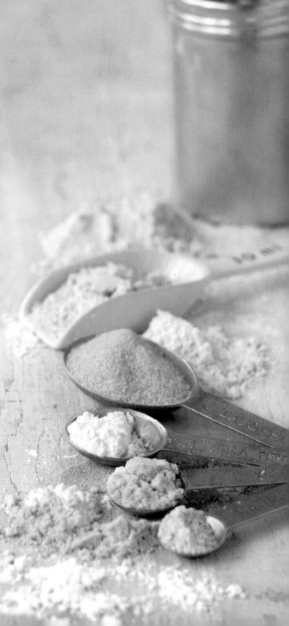

introduction

This book provides delicious ideas for gluten-free recipes, plus some alternatives to traditional family favourites that people suffering from coeliac disease, gluten intolerance or wheat allergy may miss the most.

Some recipes are inherently gluten-free and rely on fresh ingredients and creative seasonings to make them satisfying. Others require simple substitutions – when baking, for example, wheat flours are replaced with gluten-free flours, as well as chickpea/gram flour, rice flour, quinoa flour, polenta/cornmeal, tapioca and ground nuts, all of which are readily available. With this book, you'll be able to make things that taste so good that you would never know they were gluten-free. You can serve these recipes to the whole family and all of your friends and no one will notice any difference. Free-from has never tasted so good!

What is coeliac disease?

Coeliac disease is an auto-immune disease that affects the intestines, leading to poor absorption of gluten. Symptoms of coeliac disease can leave those affected feeling very unwell and lacking in energy, as well as having an upset stomach and other ailments. There is currently no cure for the condition, but it can be managed very well by changing to a diet that omits gluten products. It is important that medical advice is taken by anyone who feels they might be experiencing a sensitivity to gluten, to ascertain whether they are a coeliac or are experiencing an allergic reaction to gluten and/or wheat. Each person's symptoms are unique – some people will be able to eat some ingredients that are problematic for others. Testing is available and it is important to take steps to understand what is safe for you to eat. Sometimes coeliac disease is also coupled with other allergies and you may find that some other products, which are gluten-free, also make you unwell. A common example of this is an intolerance to dairy.

Managing a gluten-free diet

Gluten is present in varying levels in wheat, barley and rye cereals and also sometimes in oats, although this is thought to be most likely caused by cross-contamination with other cereals. Some people sensitive to gluten can eat oats and as these are a good staple ingredient in baking, some of the recipes in this book use them, but always make sure you buy brands labelled 'gluten-free'.

While it is easy to avoid products that obviously contain wheat and gluten – such as bread, cakes or pasta – there are a variety of products that contain traces of gluten, some of which are not obvious. It is not always easy to avoid such pitfalls and it is, therefore, essential to carefully check the ingredients list on product packaging to ensure that a product is gluten-free.

All forms of wheat, barley, rye and spelt must be avoided. This means that regular flours and breads are out, as well as wheat-based products, such as beer and pasta. Gluten is also commonly used by food manufacturers in a wide variety of food preparation processes, and can be found in ready-meals and other processed foods. Even a small trace of wheat used as a thickener in a sauce may make you really unwell, but always checking the labelling carefully will help you to spot unsafe ingredients.

Some of the less-obvious products that may contain gluten include:

Anti-caking agents – these are used to prevent clumping and sticking together of ingredients during food production and can contain traces of wheat. Anti-caking agents are commonly found in products such as suet but also in icing/confectioners' sugar and dried fruits.

Yeast – some dried yeasts contain wheat as a bulking agent. For safe gluten-free baking, use either fresh yeast or a gluten-free dried yeast.

Baking powder – some baking powders contain wheat. Many manufacturers are now using rice flour in place of wheat flour and so gluten-free baking powder is more commonly available in stores.

Malt products – malted drinks should all be avoided as they are wheat based, but malt extract can usually be tolerated in small amounts, for example in breakfast cereals. Malt vinegar is suitable as the protein is removed in the fermentation process and the traces left are tolerated by the vast majority of coeliacs.

Soy sauce and Worcestershire sauce – these also contain gluten so look out for gluten-free brands. Tamari soy sauce is often gluten-free.

Processed meat products – products such as sausages, sausagemeat, salamis and pâtés can contain traces of wheat, so always read the labels carefully. In recipes that call for sausagemeat, such as the Sausage Rolls on page 64, it is safest to buy gluten-free sausages and remove the meat from the skins.

Sauces, gravy powders, stocks and powdered spices – these products can sometimes be bulked out with wheat products so, again, always be sure to check the labels carefully.

Instant coffees – some contain wheat as a bulking agent. Fresh ground coffee, which can be used to make espresso or filter coffee in a machine can be used instead as these generally do not contain gluten.

Soured cream – some processes for making soured cream use wheat so it is important to use a brand that is 'pure' and gluten-free.

Avoiding contamination

One key requirement of successful gluten-free baking is to avoid cross-contamination. If you have a member of the family who is intolerant to gluten, the best solution is to remove all products containing gluten from the house. While this is the most effective way to avoid the risk of cross-contamination, it is not always practical. Where total removal is not possible, the best advice is to keep gluten-free products in sealed containers in a separate place away from products containing gluten. Label everything clearly so that there can be no confusion as to what is or isn't gluten-free.

If you have been baking with regular flour, small particles will have been released into the air during cooking, which can land on cooking equipment, surfaces and even kitchen towels and leave traces of gluten. It is therefore very important to wipe down all equipment, surfaces and utensils thoroughly and use clean cloths and aprons. Cross-contamination is also possible through using kitchen appliances and equipment, such as toasters, baking sheets and wire cooling racks. Silicone sleeves (Toastabags) can be used to shield toasters from gluten contamination. Consider investing in silicone mats that you can set aside just for gluten-free baking. If it is practical, keep separate tubs and jars of butters, spreads and preserves clearly labelled as 'gluten-free'.

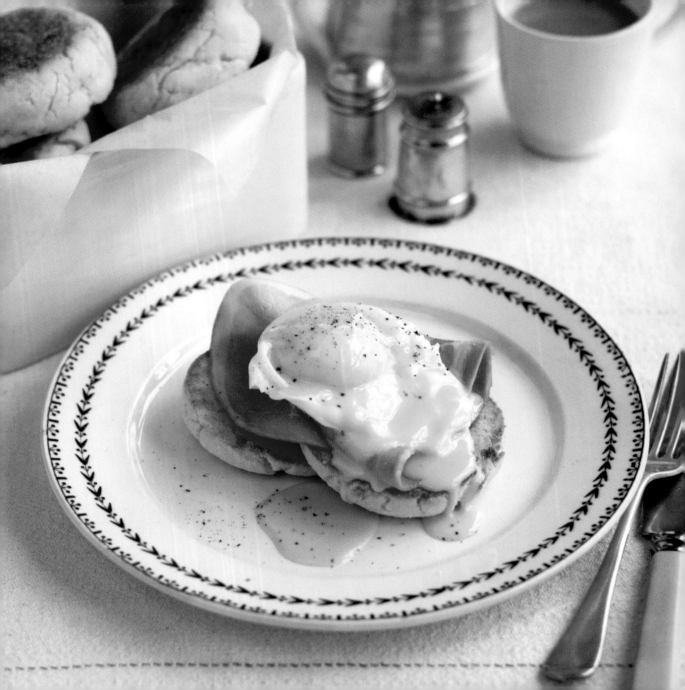

breakfast & brunch

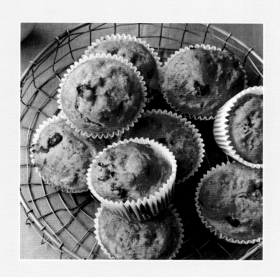

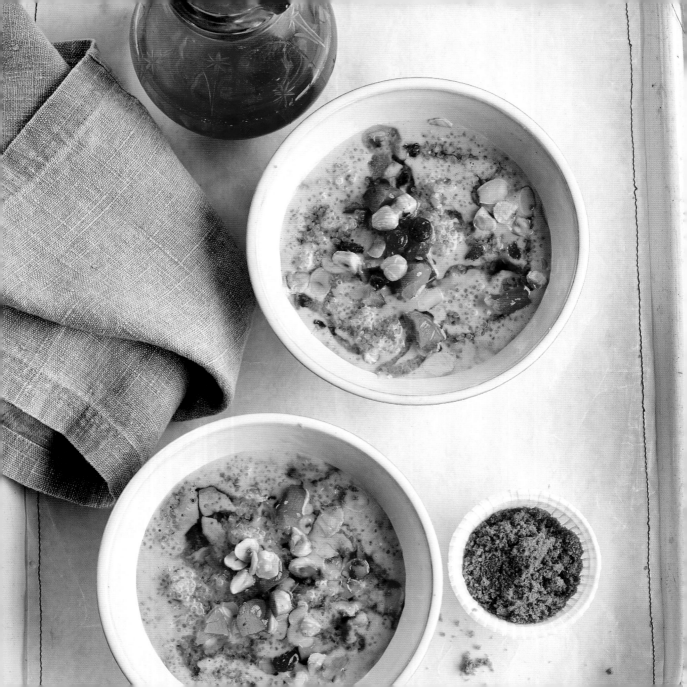

quinoa porridge with maple syrup & brown sugar

500 ml/2 cups milk, almond milk, rice milk, light coconut milk or vanilla almond milk

170 g/1 cup quinoa

¼ teaspoon sea salt

3 tablespoons soft/packed brown sugar

2 tablespoons pure maple syrup

¼ teaspoon ground cinnamon

1 teaspoon vanilla extract

chopped nuts and fruit, to serve (optional)

serves 2–4

It's time that quinoa jumped off the healthy lunch plate and into something a little sexier. Here it is led astray with maple syrup, brown sugar, vanilla and cinnamon. Who says that gluten-free can't dabble with decadence? Feel free to add bananas, raisins, berries or honey just before taking the pan off the heat.

In a medium saucepan, pour in the milk and heat over a medium heat. Stir constantly with a wooden spatula, wooden spoon or whisk. Gently scrape the bottom of the pan periodically until the milk begins to bubble and simmer, about 5–10 minutes.

When the milk simmers, add the quinoa and salt and stir until combined. Let the quinoa come to a slow boil. Cover the pan, leaving the lid slightly ajar to vent, and reduce the heat to low. Let the mixture cook on a low simmer for 10 minutes. After this time, remove the lid and stir in the brown sugar, maple syrup and cinnamon.

Place the lid loosely back on the saucepan and let the quinoa simmer on low for about 10 more minutes. Check and stir occasionally until most of the liquid is absorbed and the quinoa is tender. Reduce the heat if the quinoa appears to be simmering too quickly; add additional milk if it becomes too dry before it's tender. When done, the quinoa should look like a cross between porridge and cream of wheat. At this point, remove from the heat, add the vanilla and stir. Spoon into two big bowls or four little bowls and add chopped nuts and fruit if desired.

40 g/¼ cup red and/or yellow raspberries

45 g/¼ cup blackberries

2 tablespoons redcurrants

¼ teaspoon umeboshi vinegar

500 ml/2 cups natural plain Greek yogurt, chilled

1 banana, peeled and cubed

1 tablespoon ground flaxseeds

1 tablespoon pumpkin seeds

1 tablespoon sunflower seeds

serves 2

This is a great spring-into-summer breakfast to turn to as soon as temperatures start rising. Fresh, local, in-season fruit is more affordable than produce that is flown in from far away, so you'll be saving money, supporting local producers, eating fruit when it is at its freshest and seasonal best and, on top of all that, having a delicious and healthy morning meal!

fruit yogurt brekkie

Put the raspberries, blackberries, redcurrants and umeboshi vinegar in a bowl – the vinegar will help the berries retain their bright colours and accentuate their natural sweet taste. Crush them slightly with a fork and allow to stand for 15 minutes.

Divide the fruit mixture and chilled yogurt between two serving bowls. Add the chopped banana and all the seeds to the bowls and serve immediately.

Note

There's a whole world of fruits, seeds and nuts to choose from. Ring the changes by combining blackberries and apricots with dates and almonds; pears and prunes with sesame seeds; or peaches and grapes with raisins and hazelnuts.

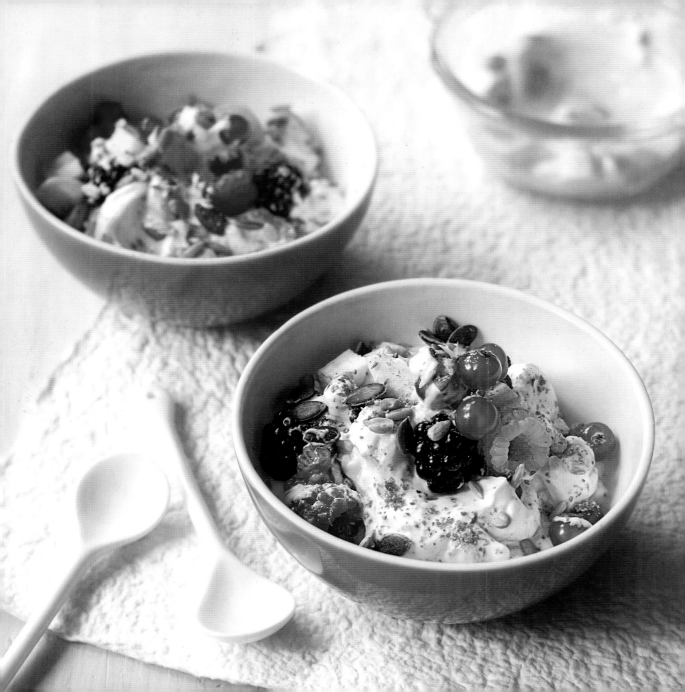

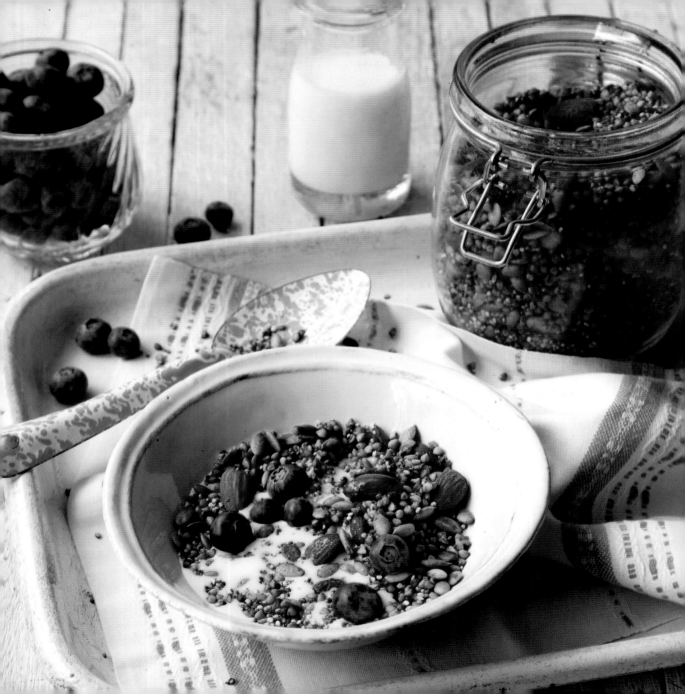

Granola is a food often associated with being healthy, but most of the time granolas contain ridiculous amounts of sugar. Even healthier versions of it can be too heavy if they are made primarily with nuts, which means you can't really have a bowl's worth of the stuff. This version contains only about 4 tablespoons of maple syrup for the entire batch (and no other added sugars in the form of dried fruits), but does contain the three most 'superfood-y' ingredients in the grain and seed category – chia seeds, buckwheat and quinoa. It has a high protein content too, since buckwheat, quinoa and chia seeds are composed of 13, 15, and 20 percent protein respectively.

power protein granola

275 g/1½ cups buckwheat groats

170 g/1 cup cooked quinoa

3 tablespoons chia seeds

35 g/¼ cup pumpkin seeds

40 g/¼ cup almonds, roughly chopped

2 teaspoons ground cinnamon

½ teaspoon grated nutmeg

1 teaspoon vanilla extract

60 ml/¼ cup coconut oil

60 ml/¼ cup pure maple syrup

3 tablespoons water (optional)

baking sheet lined with baking parchment or foil

serves 8

Preheat the oven to 180°C (350°F) Gas 4.

In a large bowl, mix the buckwheat groats, quinoa, chia seeds, pumpkin seeds, almonds, cinnamon and nutmeg.

Put the vanilla extract, coconut oil and maple syrup in a saucepan over low heat and allow to melt. Now pour it into the bowl of dry ingredients and toss to coat. Add the water if you prefer your granola a little less crunchy.

Spread the granola out on the prepared baking sheet, and don't worry if there are clumps. Bake in the preheated oven for about 1 hour.

Remove from the oven. When it has cooled for a few minutes, break it apart into clusters.

Store in a cool place in an airtight container for up to 3 weeks.

Serve with dairy-free milk and fresh fruit, such as blueberries.

coconut chia puddings

40 g/¼ cup chia seeds

1 teaspoon vanilla extract

¼ teaspoon coconut extract

1 tablespoon cashew butter

300 ml/1 ¼ cups coconut milk

1 teaspoon cinnamon

2 tablespoons shredded coconut, plus 1 tablespoon, to decorate

2 tablespoons jam, to serve (optional)

serves 2–3

There is something wonderful about taking a superfood and making a tasty (healthy) breakfast from it. Using cashew butter gives this dish a subtle warmth, but it's just as delicious when made with peanut butter.

Put the chia seeds in a large mixing bowl and set aside. Mix the rest of the ingredients together in a food processor. Then pour the mixture into the mixing bowl with the chia seeds and stir with a fork. Set aside and then stir again after 10 minutes. Divide between 2–3 glasses.

Put in the refrigerator to set. The puddings will be firm after an hour but can be left to set overnight.

When you are ready to serve, add a dollop of your favourite fruit jam and sprinkle shredded coconut over each pudding.

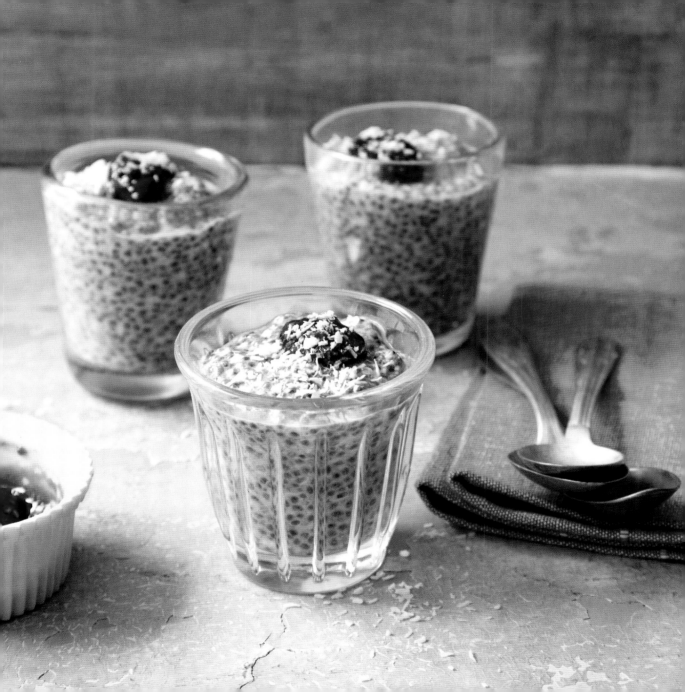

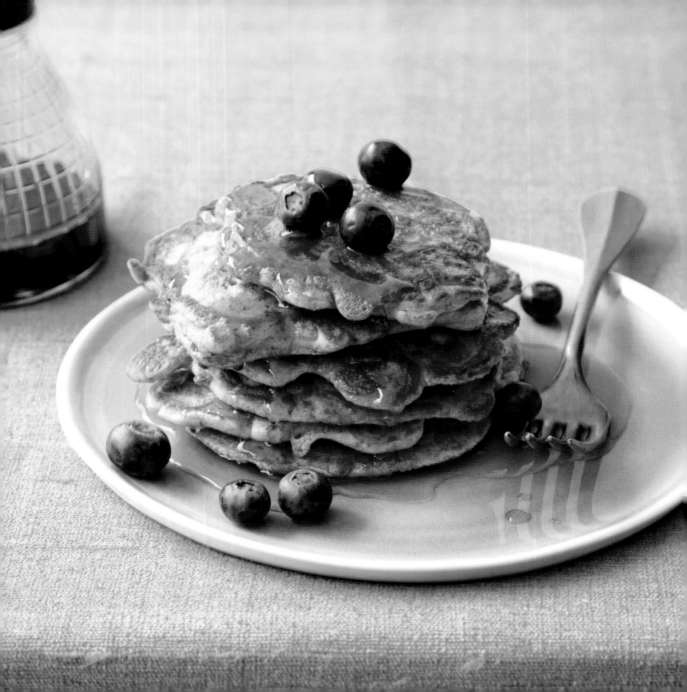

buckwheat & flaxseed pancakes

50 g/⅓ cup potato starch

½ teaspoon bicarbonate of soda/baking soda

1½ teaspoons gluten-free baking powder

70 g/½ cup buckwheat flour

60 g/½ cup brown rice flour

3 tablespoons ground flaxseeds

½ teaspoon sea salt

1 teaspoon ground cinnamon

480 ml/2 cups almond milk

2 eggs (see Note)

1 teaspoon vanilla extract

vegetable oil, for shallow frying

pure maple syrup, to taste

a handful of blueberries, to serve (optional)

serves 2–4

Pancakes with maple syrup are a popular North American breakfast favourite. In this gluten-free version, the nutrition factor is upped by adding wholegrain flours and flaxseeds in place of the usual white wheat flour. But whatever you do, don't skimp on the syrup – that's the best bit!

Sift the potato starch, bicarbonate of soda/baking soda and baking powder into a mixing bowl. Add in the remaining dry ingredients and set aside. In another bowl, combine the almond milk, eggs and vanilla extract. Add the wet into the dry ingredients gradually and whisk to a thick batter.

Heat the oil in a frying pan/skillet over a medium-high heat. Drop the batter from a spoon into the pan to form round circles. Cook until small bubbles form on the top of each pancake. Flip and cook for a further 3 minutes or until golden brown in colour.

Serve immediately, stacked on a plate and drizzled with maple syrup. Blueberries make a tasty healthy addition, if desired.

Note

If you prefer not to use eggs, you could use egg replacer or make a flax-egg mix by combining 2 tablespoons of ground flaxseeds with 6 tablespoons of water.

70 g/½ cup potato starch

1 teaspoon bicarbonate of soda/
baking soda

1 teaspoon gluten-free baking powder

1 teaspoon xanthan gum

60 g/½ cup brown rice flour

60 g/½ cup teff flour

3 tablespoons ground flaxseeds

125 g/½ cup coconut yogurt

2 eggs (see Notes)

70 ml/⅓ cup vegetable oil

70 ml/⅓ cup pure maple syrup or
agave syrup

180 ml/½ cup apple or pear purée
(available online)

1 teaspoon vanilla extract

a large handful of blueberries

*a muffin pan lined with baking
parchment or paper cases*

makes approximately 10 muffins

This is a definite contender for the best gluten-free muffin recipe ever! You can make it as a sliceable loaf cake if you prefer – simply bake the mixture in a loaf pan lined with baking parchment for 35 minutes.

dairy-free blueberry heaven yogurt muffins

Preheat the oven to 180°C (350°F) Gas 4.

Sift the potato starch, bicarbonate of soda/baking soda, baking powder and xanthan gum into a mixing bowl. Add in the remaining dry ingredients, then beat the wet ingredients into the mix, one at a time, before folding in the blueberries.

Spoon the muffin mixture into the prepared muffin pan. Bake in the preheated oven for 17 minutes or until cooked through and golden brown on top.

Serve immediately or store in an airtight container for a brunch treat.

Notes
If you'd rather not use eggs, you could use egg replacer or make a flax-egg mix by combining 2 tablespoons of ground flaxseeds with 6 tablespoons of water.

You can also substitute the apple or pear purée for store-bought fruit-flavoured baby food.

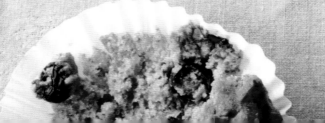

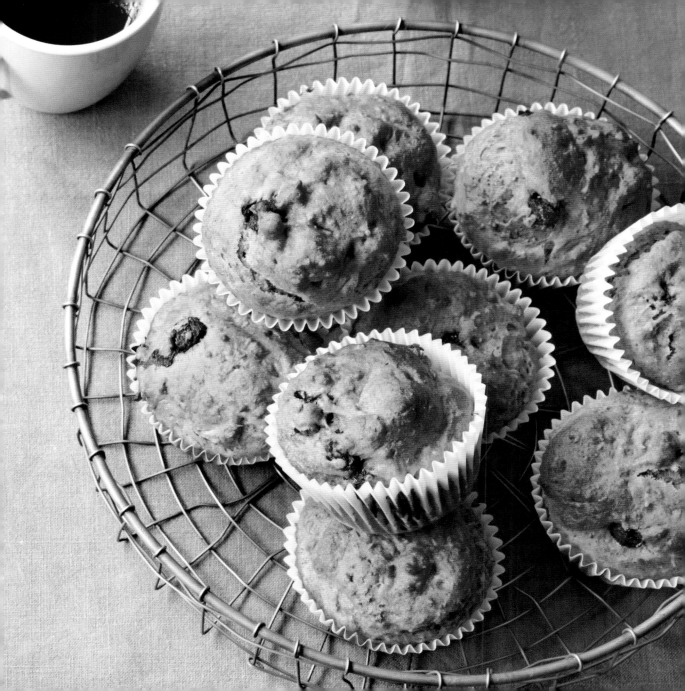

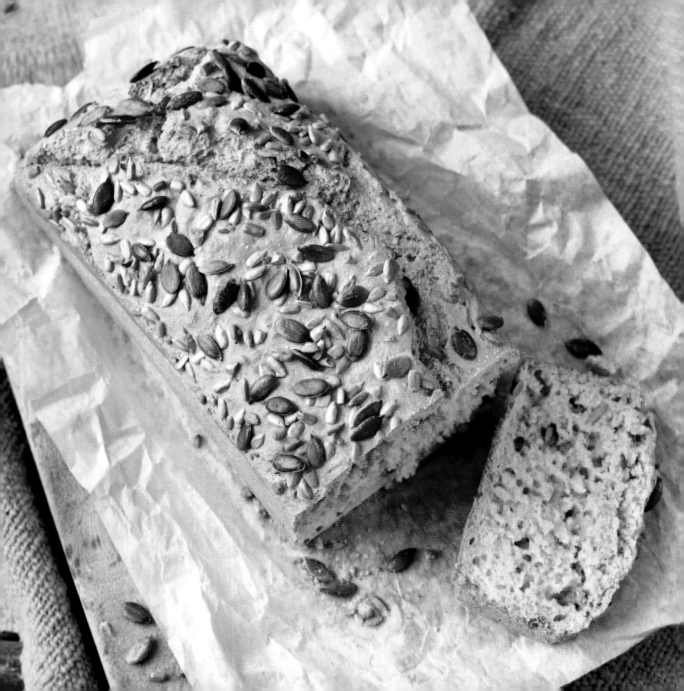

110 g/1 cup millet flakes

350 g/2½ cups millet flour

3 teaspoons gluten-free baking powder

1½ teaspoons sea salt

450 ml/1¾ cups sparkling mineral water (or gluten-free beer)

1 tablespoon olive oil

1 teaspoon apple cider vinegar

2 tablespoons seeds of your choosing (pumpkin, sesame and sunflower work well)

a 23 x 12 cm/9 x 4¾ in. loaf pan

makes 1 loaf

croutons

3 slices Seeded Loaf (see recipe above)

3 tablespoons olive oil

¼ teaspoon sea salt (or tamari)

1 teaspoon dried herbs of your choosing

a 23 x 30 cm/9 x 12 in. baking pan, well-oiled

serves 3

This lovely breakfast loaf is both gluten-free and yeast-free, so you don't need to knead it or wait for it to rise, and it stays fresh for a couple of days. It's also fantastic for making crunchy croutons to add to soups and salads.

seeded loaf

Preheat the oven to 220°C (425°F) Gas 7.

Stir together the millet flakes, flour, baking powder and salt in a bowl until well mixed. In a separate bowl, whisk together the sparkling water (or beer) with the olive oil and vinegar. Pour this into the dry ingredients, mixing vigorously with a spatula until you get a medium-thick batter.

In order to get a nicely shaped loaf, cut a sheet of baking parchment to fit inside the loaf pan without any creases. Sprinkle with 1 tablespoon of the seeds. Pour the dough into the lined pan and top with the remaining seeds. Bake in the preheated oven, reduced to 200°C (400°F) Gas 6, for 1 hour.

Remove from the oven and tip the bread out of the pan, peel off the paper and leave to cool completely on a wire rack. Wrap the bread in a dish towel and store in a cool, dry place for up to 5 days.

Variation

To make croutons, preheat the oven to 180°C (350°F) Gas 4. Cut the bread into small cubes. Mix the other ingredients in a large mixing bowl with 2 tablespoons of water and pour over the bread cubes, making sure that each one is coated. Spread the cubes out on the prepared baking pan and bake in the preheated oven for about 30 minutes, until the croutons turn golden brown and crispy. Check and stir every 5 minutes to ensure that the croutons bake evenly. Don't worry if they are a little soft when removing them from the oven – the croutons will dry out as they cool down.

pineapple bran muffins

125 g/¾ cup dried fruit (here raisins and figs)

125 g/½ cup low-fat natural/plain yogurt

60 ml/¼ cup vegetable oil

1 egg (see Note)

35 g/¼ cup potato starch

½ teaspoon bicarbonate of soda/baking soda

½ teaspoon gluten-free baking powder

½ teaspoon xanthan gum

30 g/¼ cup brown rice flour

30 g/¼ cup teff flour

2 tablespoons ground flaxseeds

105 g/¾ cup oat bran

70 g/⅓ cup sugar or sweetener

a handful of chopped pineapple

a muffin pan lined with parchment paper or paper cases

makes approximately 10 muffins

In this recipe the dried fruit is plumped up and blended, but if you need a short cut, just use store-bought organic baby food. It gives a great consistency and flavour.

Preheat the oven to 180°C (350°F) Gas 4.

Put the dried fruit in a mixing bowl and cover it with very hot but not boiling water. Leave to soak for 10 minutes, drain, and discard the water. Then purée the fruit in a food processor. If you don't have time to plump the fruit, you can substitute 125 g/½ cup of store-bought fruit-flavoured baby food.

Mix the dried fruit purée with the rest of the wet ingredients. Sift in the potato starch, bicarbonate of soda/baking soda, baking powder and xanthan gum. Then add in the remaining dry ingredients and beat until fully mixed. Lastly, fold in the chopped pineapple.

Spoon the muffin mixture into the prepared muffin pan. Bake for 20 minutes until cooked through and golden brown on top.

These can be eaten hot or cold but are really delicious served warm, straight from the oven.

Note
If you prefer not to use an egg, you could use egg replacer or make a flax-egg mix by combining 1 tablespoon of ground flaxseeds with 3 tablespoons of water.

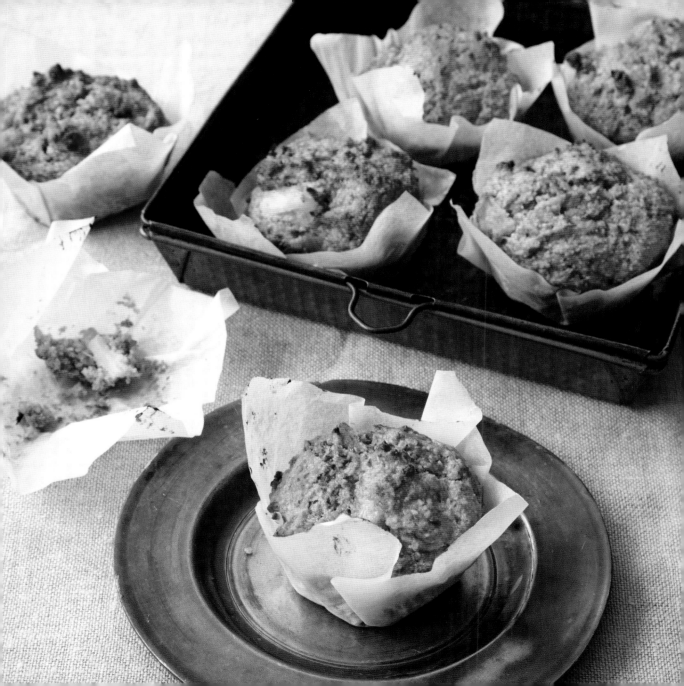

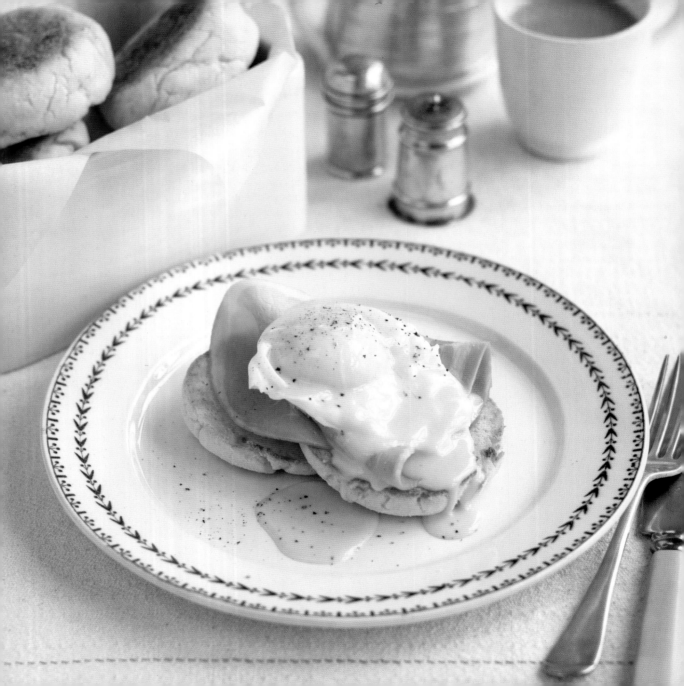

English muffins with eggs benedict

150 ml/⅔ cup warm milk

1 tablespoon easy-blend/active dried yeast

1 tablespoon caster/granulated sugar

300 g/2⅓ cups gluten-free strong white bread flour

1 teaspoon gluten-free baking powder

1 teaspoon xanthan gum

1 teaspoon sea salt

1 egg, beaten

80 ml/⅓ cup set natural/plain yogurt

60 g/4 tablespoons butter, melted and cooled, plus extra for greasing

yellow cornflour/fine cornmeal and polenta grains, for dusting

for the hollandaise

1 tablespoon white wine vinegar

freshly squeezed juice of 1–1½ lemons

1 bay leaf

1 whole egg, plus 2 egg yolks

190 g/1 stick plus 5 tablespoons butter

sea salt and freshly ground black pepper

to serve

1 teaspoon white wine vinegar

6 eggs

6 slices of thick-cut ham

serves 6

There are few finer breakfasts than a toasted muffin topped with hollandaise, poached eggs and ham: the classic Eggs Benedict.

Put the warm milk, yeast and sugar in a jug/pitcher and leave in a warm place for about 10 minutes until a thick foam has formed on top of the liquid. Sift the flour, baking powder and xanthan gum into a large mixing bowl. Add the salt, egg, yogurt, melted butter and yeast mixture, and mix well with a wooden spoon until you have a soft dough. Divide the dough into six portions. Dust a clean surface with yellow cornflour/cornmeal, roll each portion into a ball and flatten into patties, turning with your hands so that the muffin is flat on the top and bottom and has straight sides about 2.5 cm/1 inch high. Sprinkle the muffins with polenta and pat down so that it sticks to the dough, then place them on a flour-dusted baking sheet and leave, uncovered, in a warm place for 45–60 minutes. When the muffins have risen, heat a griddle pan or frying pan/skillet over a high heat. Grease the pan with a little butter and add the muffins, then turn down the heat. Cook them for about 8–10 minutes on one side, then turn over and cook the other side for a further 7–10 minutes so that they are golden brown on both sides and spring back when pressed.

To make the hollandaise, simmer the vinegar and the juice of 1 lemon in a saucepan with the bay leaf and some black pepper until the liquid has reduced by half. Remove the bay leaf and season, then pour the liquid into a food processor with the egg and egg yolks and blend together. Melt the butter in a saucepan then, motor still running, pour the warm butter into the egg mixture in a thin drizzle. Whisk until it becomes slightly thick. Taste for seasoning, adding a little lemon juice and salt and pepper if needed.

When you are ready to serve, bring a saucepan of water to the boil, add the vinegar and season. Turn down the heat so that the water is just simmering. Carefully tip the eggs one at a time into the water. Poach them for 2–3 minutes, then remove from the water with a slotted spoon.

While the eggs are cooking, cut the muffins in half and toast lightly. Top each pair of muffin halves with a slice of ham and a poached egg, spoon over some of the warm hollandaise, season and serve straight away.

1 sweet potato

extra virgin olive oil

dried chilli/hot red pepper flakes

2 red onions, sliced

handful of ripe baby plum tomatoes

2 tablespoons good balsamic vinegar

bunch of cavolo nero leaves (or
spinach)

10–12 eggs, depending on the size
of your pan

small bunch of fresh basil

1 garlic clove, peeled

sea salt and freshly ground black
pepper

*20–25-cm/8–10-inch ovenproof
frying pan/skillet or quiche dish*

serves 8–10

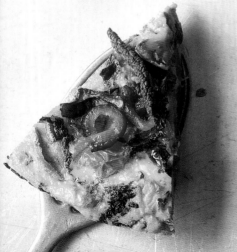

A frittata can be thrown together with whatever vegetables you
have to hand with wonderful results. Here, vibrant green cavolo
nero, orange sweet potato and red tomato vie for attention.

sweet potato, cavolo nero & plum tomato frittata with basil oil

Preheat the oven to 180°C (350°F) Gas 4.

Cut the potato in half lengthways and then into thin wedges. Toss in a
roasting pan with 2 tablespoons olive oil and a little salt, pepper and
dried chilli/red pepper flakes. Roast in the preheated oven until just
browned and starting to blister.

About 15 minutes before the sweet potato is done, toss the red onions
and tomatoes on a baking sheet with a few tablespoons of oil, the
vinegar and a sprinkling of salt and place in the oven. The skins of the
tomatoes should have just popped open and the red onions begun to
caramelize when the sweet potato is ready to take out. Leave the oven
on for the frittata.

Remove the cavolo nero leaves from their stalks and blanch in salted
boiling water for about 2 minutes. Remove and refresh with cold water.

Crack the eggs into a bowl, whisk and season well. Place the sweet
potato, cavolo nero, tomatoes and onion (reserving some for on top) in
the ovenproof frying pan/skillet or a quiche dish. Pour the beaten eggs
over and finish with the reserved vegetables on top so that you can see
their colour. Cook in the oven for 25 minutes or until the frittata has
puffed up and the top is just firm to the touch.

In the meantime, finely chop the basil and garlic and combine with
6 tablespoons olive oil to make a loose basil oil.

Allow the frittata to cool a little, then drizzle the basil oil over it and serve
with a light mixed leaf salad.

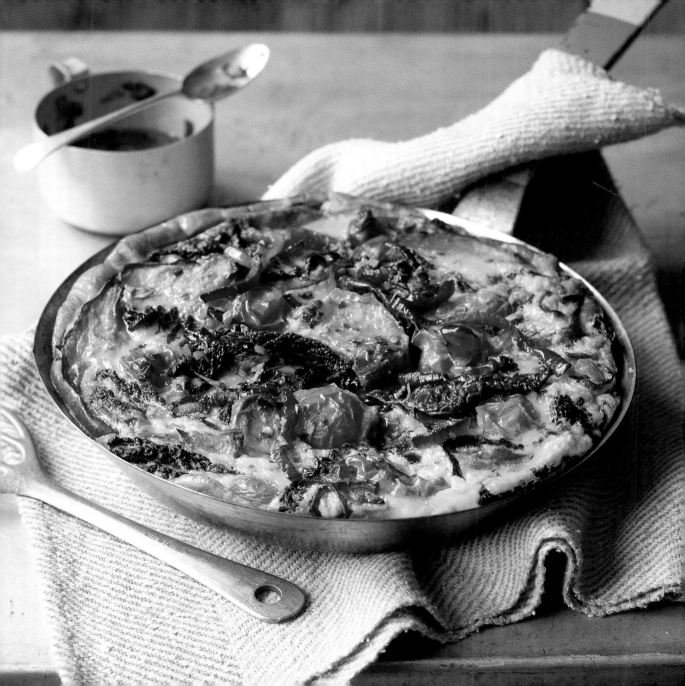

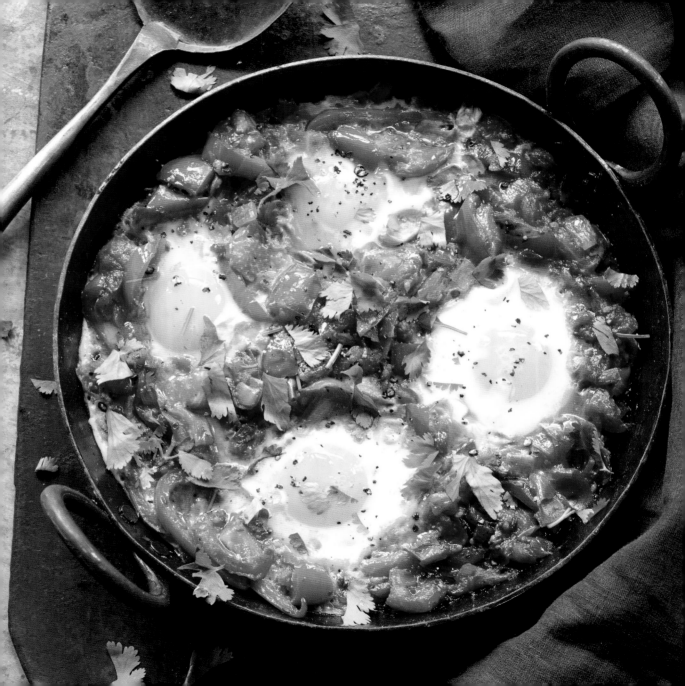

This classic North African dish makes an excellent brunch dish. Serve it with some crusty gluten-free bread for mopping up the spiced tomato sauce.

Tunisian baked eggs in tomato sauce

450 g/1 lb. ripe tomatoes

1 tablespoon olive oil

1 onion, chopped

1 red (bell) pepper, chopped into strips

1 garlic clove, chopped

1 teaspoon ground cumin

½ teaspoon harissa paste

1 teaspoon brown sugar

4 eggs

chopped fresh coriander/cilantro, to garnish

sea salt and freshly ground black pepper

serves 4

Roughly chop the tomatoes, reserving the juices.

Heat the olive oil in a large, heavy-bottomed frying pan/skillet set over a medium heat. Add the onion, (bell) pepper and garlic and fry, stirring often, for 5 minutes, until softened.

Mix together the cumin with 1 tablespoon of water in a small bowl to form a paste.

Add the harissa and cumin paste to the pan and fry, stirring, for a minute. Add the tomatoes and brown sugar, season with salt and pepper, and mix well. Bring to the boil, reduce the heat, cover and simmer for 5 minutes.

Uncover and simmer for a further 10 minutes, stirring now and then, to reduce and thicken the tomato mixture.

Break the eggs, spaced well apart, into the tomato mixture. Cover and cook over a low heat for 10 minutes until the eggs are set.

Garnish with coriander/cilantro and serve at once.

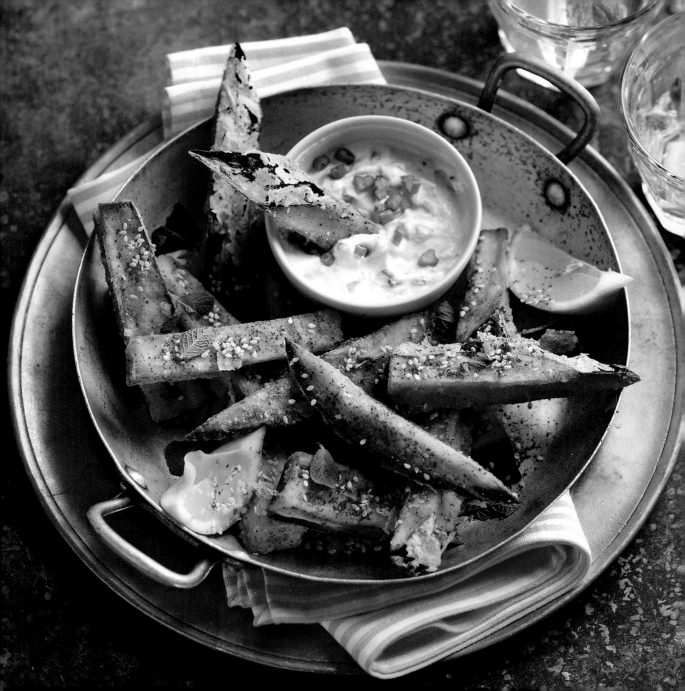

small bites & snacks

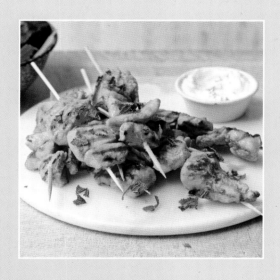

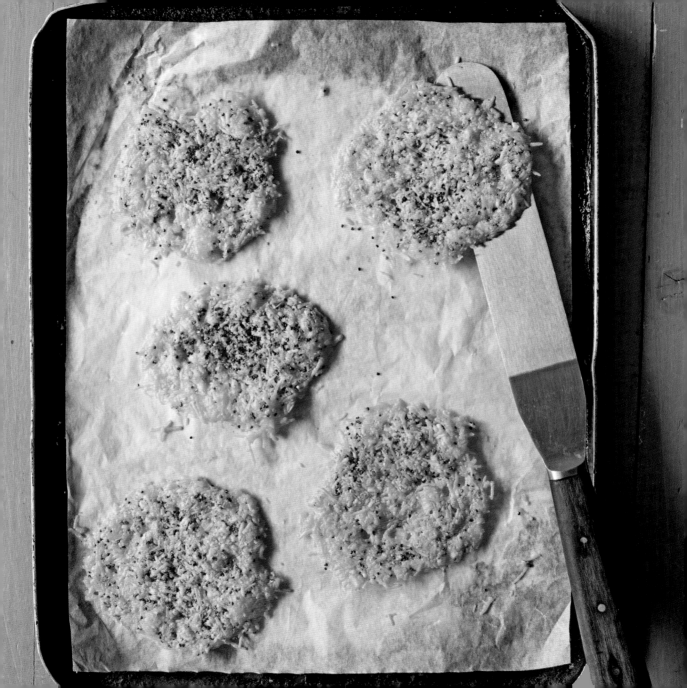

This is a lovely little recipe to have in your repertoire. With the poppy seeds they make delightfully delicate little Parmesan thins that you can serve alongside drinks and if you omit the poppy seeds, they are perfect for floating atop a bowl of French onion soup or garnishing a mushroom risotto.

Parmesan & poppy seed crisps

115 g/4 oz. Parmesan cheese, finely grated

1–2 teaspoons poppy seeds

2 baking sheets lined with non-stick baking parchment or silicone baking sheets

makes 10–12

Preheat the oven to 200°C (400°F) Gas 6.

Mix the Parmesan and poppy seeds in a small bowl, then place heaped tablespoons of the mixture onto the prepared baking sheets, well spaced apart. Gently pat down with your fingers so the mixture forms discs of around 2.5–3 cm/1–1¼ inches.

Bake in the preheated oven for 4 minutes until the cheese is bubbling and golden on top.

Remove from the oven and set the baking sheets onto wire racks to cool completely, before carefully lifting the crisps from the sheets using a palette knife to help you. Alternatively, you could cool them slightly but, while still a little warm, drape each one in turn over an upturned glass to form small baskets to serve canapés in for a party.

These crisps are best eaten on the day they are made.

Variations

If poppy seeds aren't your thing, you could omit them altogether or omit and sprinkle with freshly snipped chives just before baking. You could also try adding 1 teaspoon dried oregano or 1 teaspoon dried chilli/hot red pepper flakes in place of the poppy seeds.

olive oil crackers

200 g/1⅔ cups gluten-free plain/all-purpose flour, plus extra for dusting

1 teaspoon gluten-free baking powder

30 ml/2 tablespoons extra virgin olive oil, plus extra for brushing

to decorate

sea salt flakes and freshly ground black pepper, poppy seeds, sesame seeds, piri piri seasoning

a 6-cm/2½-inch round cookie cutter

2 baking sheets lined with non-stick baking parchment

makes about 30

These dainty crackers are a perfect nibble to serve with drinks. They can be topped with a wide variety of flavourings: here salt and pepper, poppy seeds, sesame seeds and piri piri seasoning for some extra heat are used, but you could try chopped nuts or Chinese five-spice powder, too.

Preheat the oven to 200°C (400°F) Gas 6.

Sift the flour and baking powder into a large mixing bowl. Add the olive oil and 100 ml/6 tablespoons of water and mix to a soft dough. Chill the dough in the refrigerator for 1 hour.

When chilled, roll out the dough on a flour-dusted surface until it is very thin. (It is important to use lots of flour dusted underneath and on top of the dough and also on the rolling pin, as the dough can stick easily.) Cut out about 30 circles of the dough using the cutter and place on the prepared baking sheets. Using a pastry brush, brush a generous layer of olive oil over each cracker and sprinkle with salt and pepper, poppy seeds, sesame seeds or the piri piri seasoning.

Bake the crackers in the preheated oven for 6–10 minutes until lightly golden brown. Leave to cool for a few minutes on the baking sheets, then transfer to a wire rack to cool completely.

The crackers will keep for up to 5 days in an airtight container.

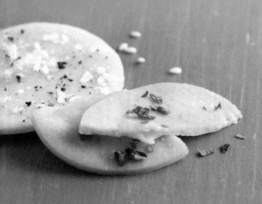

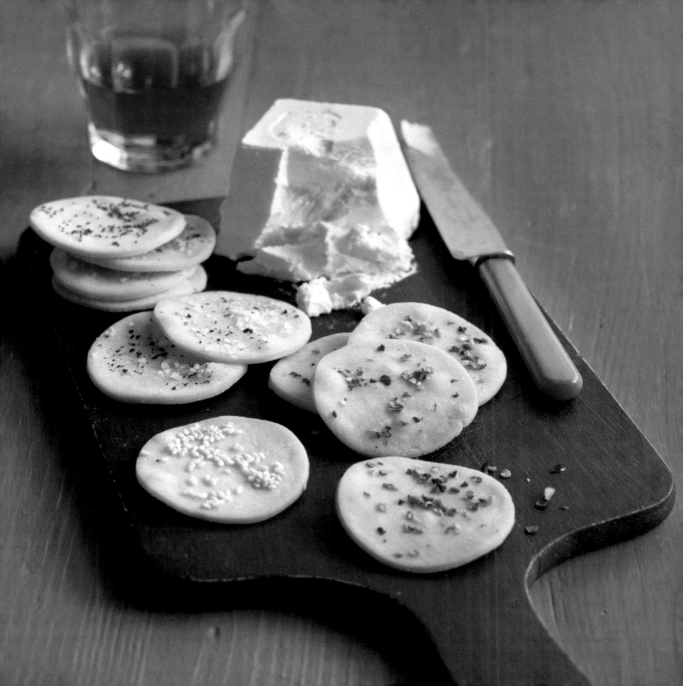

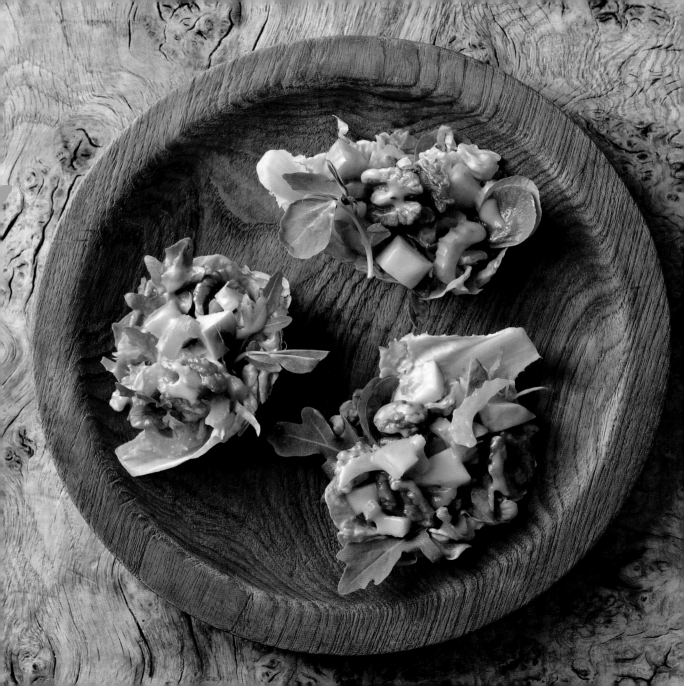

Waldorf salad wraps

2 Little Gem/Bibb lettuce heads

grated zest and freshly squeezed juice of 1 lemon

2 green dessert apples, cored and diced

100 ml/⅓ cup Mayonnaise (page 110)

6 celery sticks, sliced

150 g/1½ cups walnut halves

90 g/generous 1 cup pea shoots

60 g/generous 1 cup fresh wild rocket/arugula

serves 4

These Waldorf-style salad wraps can be served as healthy canapés or as a light meal. They are both tasty and fun to eat.

Discard a couple of the outer leaves of the lettuces and choose 12 good leaves and set them aside. Finely chop the remaining lettuce and put in a large mixing bowl.

In a separate bowl, sprinkle some lemon juice over the apple pieces and toss to coat. Add the mayonnaise, lemon zest, celery and walnut halves. Toss together to generously coat all the ingredients.

Reserve some of the pea shoots for dressing the dish, then mix together the remaining pea shoots, chopped lettuce, rocket/arugula and a squeeze of lemon juice.

To serve, place three reserved lettuce leaves on each plate; put the mixed salad on top, then the celery, apple and walnut mayonnaise on top of that. Dress with the reserved pea shoots and serve.

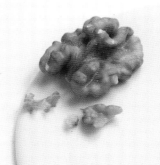

20 small open capped mushrooms

3 slices gluten-free bread

50 g/⅓ cup cranberries

1 garlic clove, peeled

1 teaspoon fresh thyme leaves

45 ml/3 tablespoons olive oil, plus extra for drizzling

sea salt and freshly ground black pepper

a few thyme flowers or small sprigs of thyme, to garnish (optional)

a baking sheet lined with non-stick baking parchment

makes 20

These pretty canapé mushrooms are topped with pretty thyme flowers (or just small sprigs of thyme). They are quick and easy to prepare and make a great nibble to serve at parties.

thyme flower mushrooms

Preheat the oven to 180°C (350°F) Gas 4.

Remove the stalks of the mushrooms and brush the caps clean with paper towels to remove any dirt. Put the mushroom caps in a roasting pan.

Put the mushroom stalks, bread, cranberries, garlic clove, thyme leaves and olive oil in a food processor and blitz to fine crumbs, then season with salt and pepper. Place a spoonful of the crumbs into each mushroom cap and drizzle with extra olive oil.

Bake the mushrooms in the preheated oven for 15–20 minutes, until the crumbs are crisp and the mushrooms softened. Sprinkle with thyme flowers or a few small sprigs of thyme, to garnish, and serve warm.

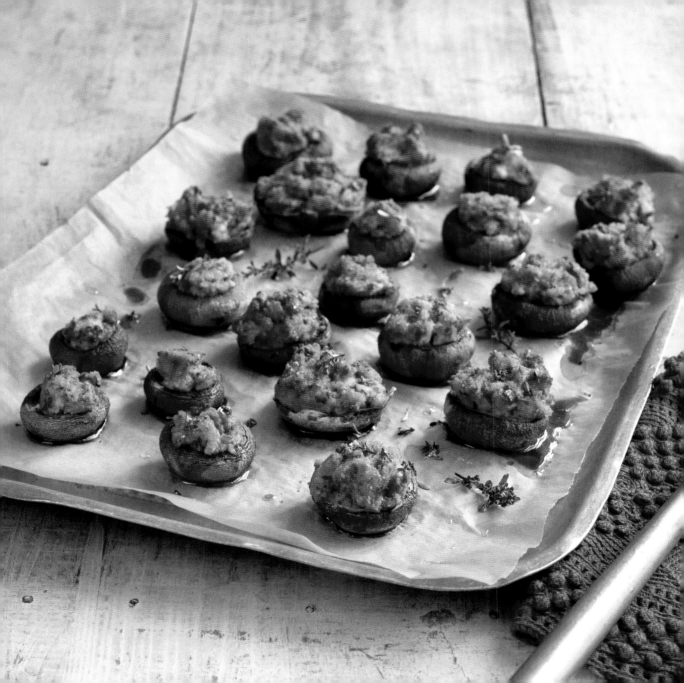

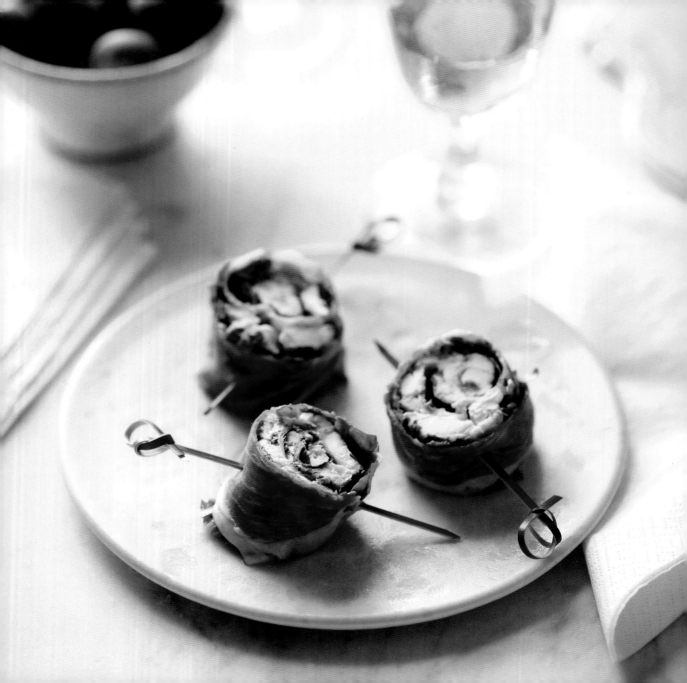

12 slices Parma ham/prosciutto

3 tablespoons Puttanesca Relish (see recipe below)

a handful of rocket/arugula (about 4–5 leaves per roll)

200 g/7 oz. goats' cheese, sliced into 12 strips (or cheese of your choice; Gorgonzola is good too)

makes 24

for the puttanesca relish

55 g/2 oz. pitted black or Kalamata olives

2 canned anchovy fillets, drained

2 teaspoons capers, drained

a big pinch of freshly chopped coriander/cilantro

½ garlic clove, peeled

1 tablespoon olive oil

200-g/7-oz. can tomatoes, drained (you don't want too much liquid)

sea salt and freshly ground black pepper

makes 1 small jar

Sushi was another triumph in man's battle against shelflife. Like salumi, the method of fermenting fish with rice and vinegars was designed to extend the life of the fish. Before methods were developed to make the rice and wrapping just as delicious as the fish in the middle, the rice was discarded before the fish was eaten. So, as a tribute to our ancestors' peers in the Far East, here's a sushi-inspired recipe using charcuterie.

'sushi-style' prosciutto-wrapped goats' cheese & rocket

First make the puttanesca relish. Pop all the ingredients into a food processor and whizz until the texture is relatively smooth but stop before it becomes more like a purée. Transfer the mixture to a 200 g/7 oz. sterilized jar or an airtight container, or divide it between two ramekins and cover. It will keep for a week or two in a sealed container in the refrigerator. It is also suitable for freezing. If you do freeze it, defrost it slowly in the refrigerator and then taste before you serve it, topping up any of the flavours that you think it needs.

Lay a slice of Parma ham/prosciutto flat on a board or plate. Spread 1 teaspoon of the relish over the surface. Sprinkle 4–5 rocket/arugula leaves on the top, then put a strip of cheese on top in the middle.

Roll the Parma ham/prosciutto over on itself to enclose the filling, like a 'nori roll', and then slice (it is easiest to snip with kitchen scissors) in half to create two circles. Push a cocktail stick/toothpick through each assembled bite to hold it together. Repeat to make 24 bites in total. Serve immediately.

cornichons wrapped in salami

12 slices salami

12 cornichons (or 12 small slices of pickled gherkin)

freshly ground black pepper

makes 12

As simple as the name suggests. These mini gherkins are often served with salami because the flavours complement each other perfectly. This combination really is a delight for the taste buds — saltiness from the meat and acidity of the pickled cornichons.

For each bite, just wrap a slice of salami around a cornichon and pop a cocktail stick/toothpick through the middle to hold them together.

Repeat to make 12 bites in total. Crack a little pepper over the plate and serve.

mozzarella pearls/balls wrapped in prosciutto

3 slices Parma ham/prosciutto

12 mini mozzarella pearls/balls

freshly ground black pepper

makes 12

So simple, just like the recipe above. A whole slice of Parma ham/prosciutto per mini mozzarella pearl/ball would make a heavy mouthful, as well as being expensive for entertaining, so cut each slice of Parma ham/prosciutto into quarters.

Cut each slice of Parma ham/prosciutto lengthways into quarters (kitchen scissors are best for doing this) to make 12 strips in total. Wrap each strip around a mini mozzarella pearl/ball.

Pop a cocktail stick/toothpick through the middle of each assembled bite to hold it together, crack a little black pepper over the plate and serve.

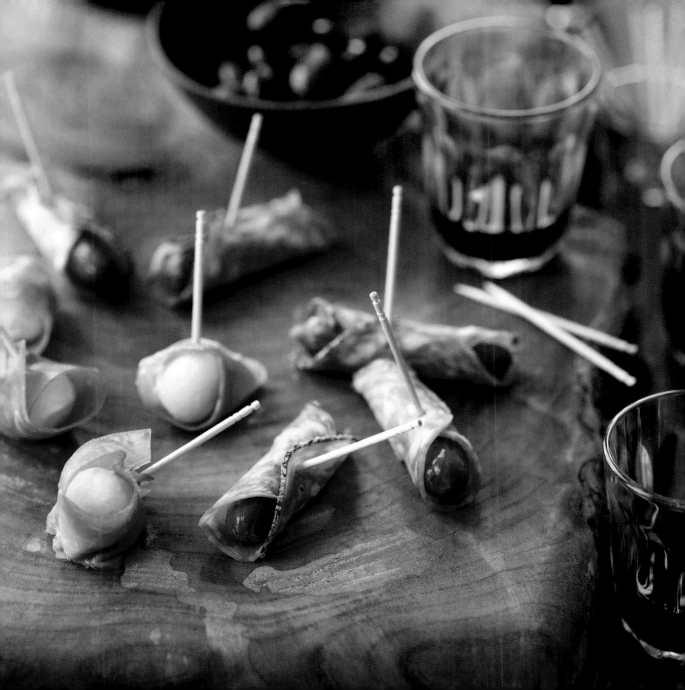

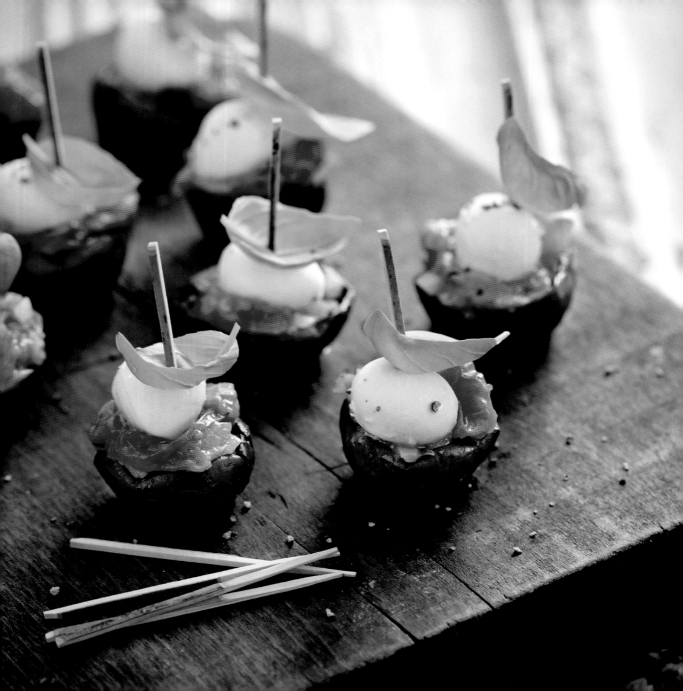

aubergine/eggplant & tomato toothpicks

10 baby aubergines/eggplants (or
1 long, thin aubergine/eggplant)

3 tablespoons extra virgin olive oil

1 tablespoon fresh thyme leaves

2 tablespoons finely grated Parmesan
cheese

20 mini mozzarella pearls/balls

sea salt and freshly ground black
pepper

small fresh basil leaves, to garnish

for the tomato sauce

3–4 tablespoons extra virgin olive oil

1 white onion, finely chopped

2 garlic cloves, finely chopped

400 g/14 oz. ripe cherry tomatoes,
halved

100 ml/⅓ cup white wine

1 teaspoon white sugar

a small handful of torn fresh basil

makes 20

Baby aubergines/eggplants are perfect for this recipe, and look so pretty – but if you can't get hold of them, simply choose one that is longer rather than very round.

Preheat the oven to 190°C (375°F) Gas 5.

If you are using baby aubergines/eggplants, simply cut them in half. If you are using a large aubergine/eggplants, cut it in half lengthways, then into wedges that create small 'boats'. You will have to cut a little from the top of each wedge to create a flat surface. Score the surface without the skin of each with a criss-cross pattern.

Brush the aubergine/eggplant with extra virgin olive oil, season with salt and pepper, scatter with thyme leaves, then sprinkle over the Parmesan. Arrange on a baking sheet and cook in the preheated oven for about 20 minutes or so, until the aubergine/eggplant is soft and the skin is crisp.

Meanwhile, make the tomato sauce. Heat the oil in a large frying pan/skillet over a low-medium heat and cook the onion and garlic for about 15 minutes, until softened but not coloured. Add the cherry tomatoes and the wine. Stir in the sugar, season with salt and pepper and let the mixture bubble gently for about 20 minutes. Add the torn basil, and leave to bubble for another 10 minutes or so, until the sauce is thick and sticky.

Spoon a little of the sauce onto each piece of aubergine/eggplant, top with a mozzarella pearl/ball and garnish with a small basil leaf, securing everything with a cocktail stick/toothpick. Serve immediately.

100 g/3½ oz. walnut pieces or halves

1 teaspoon freshly chopped rosemary

½ teaspoon finely grated lemon zest

1 tablespoon olive oil

1 teaspoon caster/granulated sugar

100 g/½ cup cream cheese

85 g/3 oz. Gorgonzola Dolce or other creamy blue cheese

60 ml/¼ cup soured cream

sea salt and freshly ground black pepper

celery sticks, green apple wedges or gluten-free breadsticks, to serve

serves 4–6

If you prefer a really strong blue cheese, replace the Gorgonzola Dolce with stilton or another hard blue cheese and blitz together with the soured cream in a blender until smooth before adding to the dip.

blue cheese & walnut dip

Preheat the oven to 180°C (350°F) Gas 4.

Put the walnuts, rosemary and lemon zest in a baking pan and drizzle with the olive oil. Sprinkle over the sugar and season with salt and pepper. Shake the pan so that all the nuts are coated in the oil and herbs. Bake for about 5 minutes until the nuts are hot, taking care that they do not burn. Remove from the oven and leave to cool.

Blitz three-quarters of the walnuts in a food processor or blender. Tip the ground nuts into a bowl with the cream cheese, blue cheese and soured cream and whisk together until smooth and creamy with a slight nutty crunch. Season to taste. Spoon the dip into a bowl and sprinkle over the remaining roasted nuts.

Serve with celery sticks, apple wedges or breadsticks, as preferred.

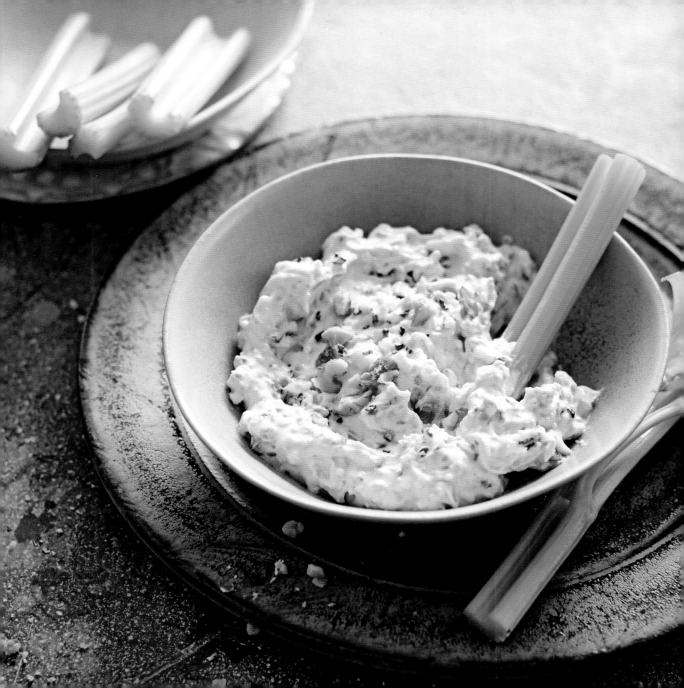

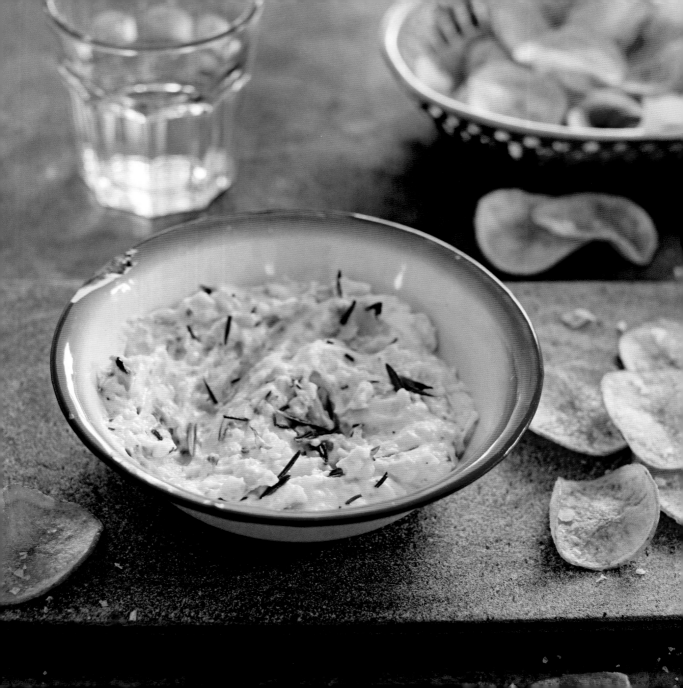

When onions are roasted, they develop a sweet and delicious caramel flavour, perfect for this tangy smoky dip which is something of a retro classic. Here it is served with deliciously light and crunchy home-made potato crisps/chips.

French onion dip with potato crisps/chips

4 medium brown onions

5 sprigs fresh thyme

2 tablespoons olive oil

250 g/9 oz. cream cheese, at room temperature

3 tablespoons crème fraîche

sea salt and freshly ground black pepper

potato crisps/chips (see below) or crackers, to serve

for the potato crisps/chips

800 g/1¾ lb. small waxy fingerling potatoes, such as Anya, Pink Fir Apple or Kipfler

125 ml/½ cup olive oil

125 ml/½ cup vegetable oil

serves 6

Preheat the oven to 180°C (350°F) Gas 4.

Peel the onions and cut them into quarters. Put the onions in a roasting pan, add the thyme sprigs and drizzle with the olive oil. Season well with salt and pepper and bake in the preheated oven for 30–40 minutes until the onions are soft and have started to caramelize. Give them a stir towards the end of cooking so they don't burn. Remove from the oven and leave to cool. Discard any onions that have gone black as they will make the dip bitter.

Remove the thyme sprigs and run your fingers along them to remove the leaves, reserving one sprig for garnish, if you wish. Add the leaves, and onions in their cooking juices, to a blender and blitz to a smooth purée.

Whisk the cream cheese into the crème fraîche and blend with the onion purèe. Taste for seasoning, adding more salt and pepper if needed.

To make the potato crisps/chips, cut the potatoes into slices about 3 mm/⅛ in. thick. Bring a large saucepan of lightly salted water to the boil. Add the potatoes, cover the pan and remove from the heat. Leave in the hot water for 5 minutes. Drain well and arrange the slices on a wire rack in a single layer until completely cool. Put the oils in a saucepan or large frying pan/skillet set over a high heat. When the oil is hot, cook the potato slices in batches for 5–6 minutes each, turning once or twice, until crisp and golden. Remove from the oil using a metal slotted spoon and drain on paper towels.

Spoon the dip into a bowl and garnish with the reserved thyme leaves. Serve with the warm potato crisps/chips or crackers, for dipping.

chorizo & scallop skewers

This is as lovely a combination of textures as it is of flavours. The scallops become slightly pink with the chorizo oil, and the taste of paprika permeates the soft flesh. Frozen scallops cook beautifully and chorizo has a lovely long shelf life, so this combination is easy to have on hand for all sorts of useful recipes – from canapés and stews to salads and risottos.

12 shelled scallops (or frozen scallops, defrosted)

olive oil, for frying

12 x 1-cm/½-inch cubes gluten-free chorizo

freshly ground black or pink pepper

paprika, for sprinkling

makes 12

First fry the scallops in a little olive oil in a frying pan/skillet over a high heat for 1 minute on each side, until cooked. Add a good scrunch of pepper, then add the chorizo cubes and fry for a further 2–3 minutes, turning and stirring everything often.

Remove the chorizo and scallops from the pan, and leave until cool enough to handle, then thread one scallop and chorizo cube onto a cocktail stick/toothpick. Put the scallop on first as the chorizo does a better job of gripping the stick.

Repeat to make 12 canapés in total. Serve immediately, while still warm, sprinkled with a little paprika, if you like.

Variation
You can always add a little chilli/chili powder or paprika to coat the scallops before cooking, but you may find that enough flavourful oil comes out of good-quality chorizo as you fry it.

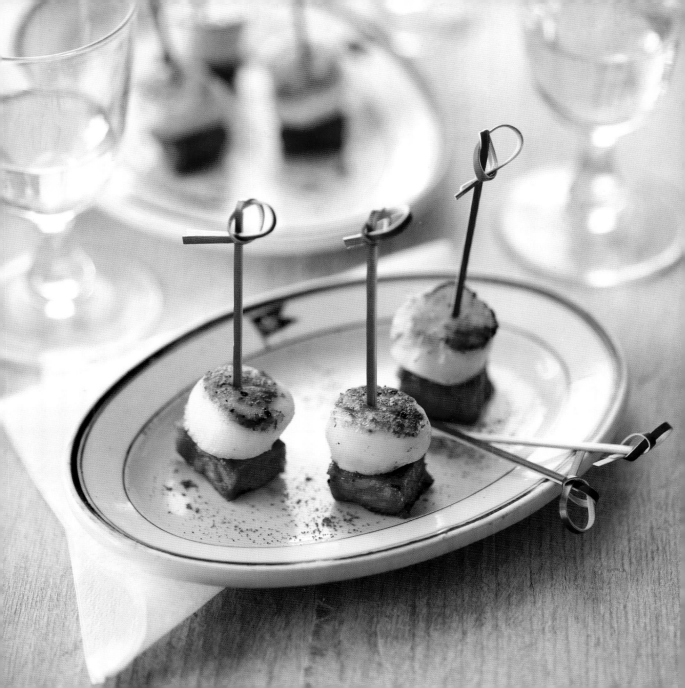

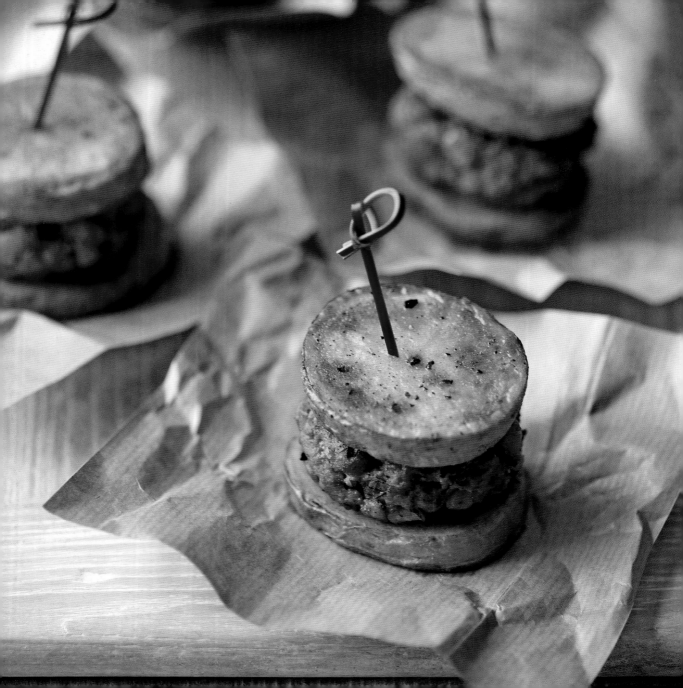

pork & apple sliders

A 'slider' is a mini burger and it makes a great canapé for entertaining and is a lovely choice for children's plates. This gluten-fee version uses fried potato discs instead of the usual mini bread rolls.

10 g/2 teaspoons butter

50 g/½ cup finely diced dessert or cooking apple

180 g/6 oz. really good pork mince/ground pork

10 g/2 teaspoons dried gluten-free breadcrumbs

10 g/2 teaspoons tomato purée/paste

a pinch of freshly chopped parsley

sea salt and freshly ground black pepper, to season

for the potato 'buns'

4 new potatoes

10 g/2 teaspoons butter

makes 4

Heat the butter in a frying pan/skillet over a medium heat and fry the diced apple pieces for about 6 minutes until they brown and start to go sticky. Remove the apple from the pan and set on a plate to cool (you can chill a plate in the fridge before you start to help speed this up). Set aside the pan – you'll use it again later.

Mix the pork mince/ground pork with a pinch of salt, the breadcrumbs, tomato purée/paste and parsley really well in a bowl. Add the apple pieces once they've cooled a bit and mix. Divide the mixture in half and then in half again to get four even pieces (each weighing approximately 55 g/2 oz.). Shape and flatten each portion – flatter sliders are easier to cook and serve.

Meanwhile, for the potatoes, bring a pan of water to the boil. Leave the skins on the new potatoes and slice them approximately 1 cm/½ inch thick. You need two slices per slider, but make 12 slices to be on the safe side (you can always nibble them while the sliders are cooking later). Add the potato slices to the boiling water and parboil them for just 2 minutes to soften. Drain and set aside.

Heat the butter in the pan from earlier over a medium heat and pick out the best-looking potato slices to fry with a good crack of black pepper. Cook well and then set aside on a wire rack or paper towel, with the slices not touching each other to keep them crispy.

Add the sliders to the same pan and fry for 3–4 minutes on each side, until cooked through.

To serve, put a slider between two potato slices and use a cocktail stick/toothpick to keep the slider together, then serve.

a generous pinch of saffron threads

2 garlic cloves, peeled

3 tablespoons olive oil, plus extra for basting

freshly squeezed juice of ½ lemon

500 g/1 lb. 2 oz. chicken breast fillets, cut into approx. 2.5-cm/1-inch cubes

sea salt

torn fresh mint leaves, to garnish

8 wooden skewers, soaked in water

serves 4

for the tzatziki

½ cucumber

1 garlic clove, crushed

250 g/1½ cups natural/plain Greek yogurt

1 tablespoon freshly chopped mint leaves

1 tablespoon olive oil

1 teaspoon white wine vinegar

salt

serves 6

Marinating chicken is a simple but effective way of adding flavour. These kebabs/kabobs would also be great for a barbecue. Serve with basmati rice, the Tzatziki dip (below) or a raita and a side salad.

saffron garlic chicken kebabs/kabobs

Grind the saffron threads, then soak in 1 teaspoon of warm water.

Pound the garlic into a paste and mix with a pinch of salt.

Mix together the garlic, saffron water, olive oil, lemon juice and more salt in a large bowl to make the marinade. Add the chicken pieces and toss, coating thoroughly in the marinade. Cover and marinate in the fridge for 4–6 hours, turning over the chicken pieces halfway through.

To make the tzatziki, peel the cucumber and grate it. Sprinkle with salt and set aside for 15 minutes to draw out moisture; rinse and drain and pat dry with paper towels. Mix together the grated cucumber, garlic, yogurt, chopped mint, olive oil and vinegar. Cover and chill until ready to serve.

Preheat the grill/broiler until very hot. Thread the marinated chicken onto the skewers, dividing the pieces evenly.

Grill the chicken kebabs/kabobs for about 15 minutes until cooked through and the juices run clear, turning often and basting with a little oil if required. Garnish with torn fresh mint and serve at once with the tzatziki.

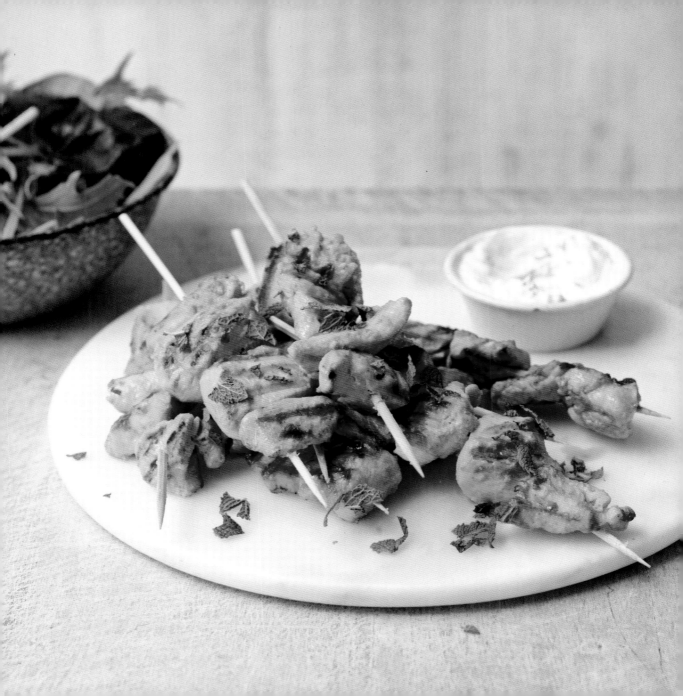

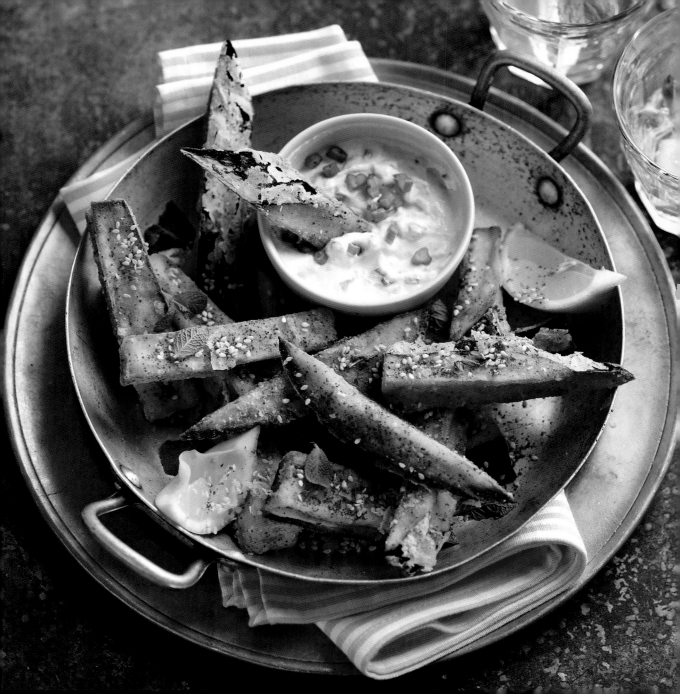

500 g/1 lb. 2 oz. aubergines/eggplants, ends trimmed and cut into 2-cm/¾-in. wide strips

125 g/1 cup rice flour

1 tablespoon sumac, plus extra to serve

2–3 sprigs fresh mint, leaves stripped and very finely chopped

1 teaspoon fine sea salt

1 tablespoon toasted sesame seeds

vegetable oil, for frying

a few fresh mint leaves and lemon wedge, to serve

for the lemon & tahini dip

200 g/7 oz. natural/plain Greek yogurt

3 tablespoons tahini

1 garlic clove, crushed

freshly squeezed juice of ½ lemon

1 spring onion/scallion, finely chopped

1 teaspoon toasted sesame seeds

clear honey, for drizzling

pomegranate molasses, for drizzling

serves 2 or 4 as a side

The velvety smooth texture of aubergine/eggplant is the perfect vehicle for some wonderful Middle Eastern ingredients: sesame seeds, mint, sumac and lemon. Zingy, zesty and fresh, serve this at lunch with a selection of salads or with scrambled eggs for a new twist on brunch.

aubergine/eggplant & sumac fries

A few hours before serving (ideally 2–12 hours), put the aubergine/eggplant strips in a large bowl and add cold water and some ice to cover. Set a plate on top to weigh the aubergine/eggplant down; it must stay submerged.

Meanwhile, make the lemon and tahini dip. In a bowl, stir together the yogurt, tahini, garlic, lemon juice and most of the spring onion/scallion. Sprinkle over the sesame seeds and top with a drizzle each of honey and pomegranate molasses and the remaining spring onion/scallion.

When ready to cook the fries, combine the rice flour, sumac, chopped mint and salt in a shallow bowl and mix well.

Fill a large saucepan one-third full with the oil or, if using a deep-fat fryer, follow the manufacturer's instructions. Heat the oil to 190°C (375°F) or until a cube of bread browns in 30 seconds.

Working in batches, transfer the damp aubergine/eggplant to the rice flour mixture and coat lightly. Place in a frying basket and lower into the hot oil carefully. Fry until golden, 3–4 minutes. Remove and drain on paper towels. Repeat until all of the aubergine/eggplant has been fried.

Mound on a platter and scatter over the sesame seeds, some sumac and the mint leaves. Serve with lemon wedges and the lemon and tahini dip.

fresh broad/fava bean falafels

350 g/2⅓ cups shelled fresh broad/fava beans

½ small bunch fresh mint, leaves only

½ small bunch fresh parsley, leaves only

2 garlic cloves, crushed

½ teaspoon sea salt

¼ teaspoon cumin seeds, crushed

1 teaspoon ground coriander

1 tablespoon chickpea/gram flour

250 ml/1 cup vegetable oil, for frying

serving suggestion

baked pumpkin squares

pink or regular sauerkraut

rocket/arugula or microgreens

Mayonnaise (see page 110)

makes 10 falafels

The most important step in making these falafels is to blend all the ingredients really well into a thick paste. Chunky falafel mix burns easily and tends to fall apart during frying. The aim is for these pointed falafels to get a nice crunchy crust with a juicy, bright-green inside. You can use fresh or thawed peas instead of broad/fava beans, with equally yummy results.

Bring a pan of water to the boil and boil the broad/fava beans for 1 minute. Drain and run them under cold water to cool them down to the point where you can handle them. Pinch their skins off with your fingers and slip the inner bright green beans out. You should get about 250 g/1½ cups peeled beans.

In a food processor fitted with an 'S' blade, chop the mint and parsley, then add the skinned beans and whizz until chopped into a paste. Scoop into a bowl, add all the remaining ingredients (except the frying oil) and knead for a second to incorporate.

Scoop up a small amount of mixture and use two spoons to shape into oval balls with lightly pointed ends. Deep-fry in hot oil for 3–4 minutes or until nicely browned.

Serve these falafels in wide bowls, placed alongside baked pumpkin, pink or regular sauerkraut and rocket/arugula or microgreens, and drizzled with mayonnaise. A very satisfying and nutritious meal!

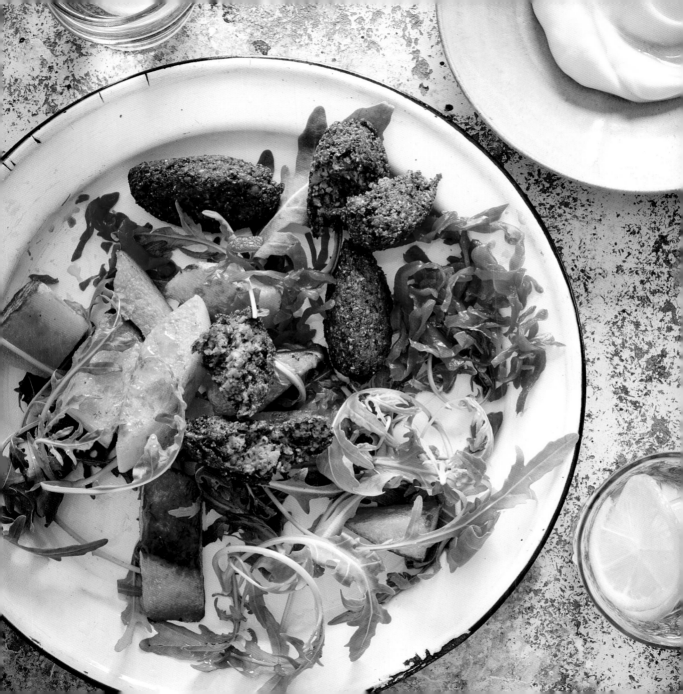

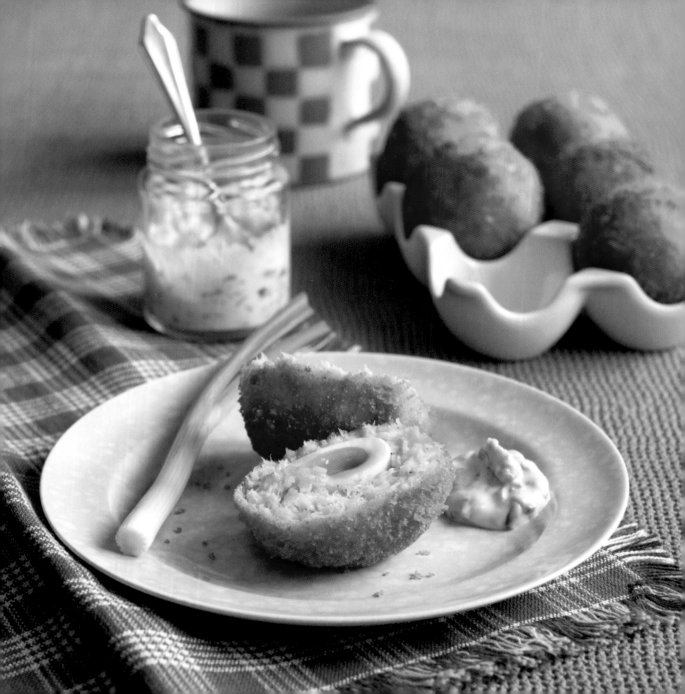

smoked haddock Scotch eggs

8 quails' eggs

500 ml/2 cups milk

1 garlic clove, thinly sliced

150 g/5½ oz. potatoes, peeled and quartered

1 sprig fresh thyme

250 g/9 oz. undyed smoked haddock, deboned

4 slices gluten-free bread

3–4 tablespoons gluten-free plain/all-purpose flour

2 eggs, beaten

sea salt and freshly ground black pepper

vegetable oil, for frying

makes 8

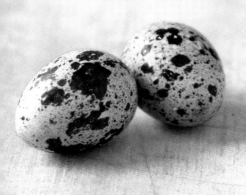

Rather than the sausagemeat traditionally used in Scotch eggs, these quails' eggs are wrapped in smoked haddock, then coated in crispy gluten-free breadcrumbs. They make a great picnic snack, or an accompaniment to smoked haddock chowder.

Bring a pan of water to the boil and gently lower the quails' eggs in. Cook for 2½ minutes, then drain the eggs and submerge in cold water to stop them cooking. Once cool, peel the eggs and set aside.

Put the milk and garlic in a saucepan and bring to the boil. Add the potatoes and thyme and poach for 15–20 minutes over a gentle heat until the potatoes are just soft. Add the fish to the pan and poach for 10–15 minutes until cooked through. Take the pan off the heat and remove just the fish. Remove the skin and any bones from the fish.

Once the potatoes have cooled in the liquid, drain, reserving a little of the milk. Remove the thyme sprig, then mash the potatoes. Flake the fish into the potato and mix everything together well. If the mixture is too dry, add a little of the poaching milk. Season with black pepper and a little salt.

Lay a piece of clingfilm/plastic wrap on a clean flat surface. Place a large spoonful of the potato mixture in the centre of the clingfilm/plastic wrap and press out thinly with the back of a spoon. Place a quail's egg in the centre of the potato and use the clingfilm/plastic wrap to pull the potato up and around to cover the whole egg. Remove the clingfilm/plastic wrap and shape into a ball in your hands. Set aside while you repeat the process with the remaining eggs and potato, then chill in the refrigerator for at least 30 minutes.

Blitz the bread to fine crumbs in a food processor, then tip into a bowl. Put the flour in another bowl and the beaten eggs in a third. Heat the oil in a saucepan until it is hot enough to make a breadcrumb dropped into it sizzle. Roll a haddock ball in the flour to give it a light dusting, then roll it in the beaten egg and finally in the breadcrumbs to coat. Repeat to coat all of the balls. Add the eggs to the oil pan in batches and cook for about 2–3 minutes until they are golden brown, turning halfway through.

These mini sausage rolls are made with hot water pastry, which is easier to roll than shortcrust. You can also use beef, lamb or venison sausagemeat, or a vegetarian filling of cheese and onion.

sausage rolls

350 g/12 oz. sausagemeat (if you can't find gluten-free sausagemeat, remove the skins from gluten-free sausages, which are readily available)

2 tablespoons freshly chopped parsley

1 teaspoon freshly ground black or white pepper

1 batch Hot Water Pastry (see page 67), refrigerated

1 egg, beaten

wholegrain mustard, to serve

a baking sheet lined with non-stick baking parchment

makes 16

Preheat the oven to 190°C (375°F) Gas 5.

In a bowl, or using a food processor on pulse setting, mix together the sausagemeat, parsley and pepper with 2 tablespoons of water until completely combined.

Take the pastry from the fridge and lightly knead on a clean, cool work surface. Lay a piece of clingfilm/plastic wrap onto the work surface. Place the pastry ball in the middle and lay a second piece of clingfilm/plastic wrap over the top. Roll out the pastry quite thinly in an oblong shape. The thickness should be only around 2–3 mm/⅛ inch.

Remove the top layer of clingfilm/plastic wrap and cut down the middle of the pastry lengthways so that you have two long rectangles. Place the sausagemeat in a thin roll running the length of the two pastry pieces – half of the sausagemeat on each.

Brush the long edge of one of the pastry pieces with the beaten egg, then gently lift and roll the pastry over the sausage filling, pressing it onto itself at the other side to form a tight seal. Trim the excess away and then roll the whole thing carefully so that it is cylindrical in shape and the seal is at the bottom. Repeat with the other pastry and filling.

Using a sharp knife, cut each roll into eight pieces, or more if you want really tiny sausage roll bites, then arrange on the prepared baking sheet.

Brush the tops with the remaining beaten egg and bake in the preheated oven for 12 minutes. If the sausage rolls are not yet golden and the sausage cooked through, return to the oven for a few more minutes. Remove from the oven and cool slightly before serving with wholegrain mustard on the side. They are best eaten on the day they are made, but can be prepared in advance and stored, uncooked, in the fridge, covered with clingfilm/plastic wrap, baking just before you need to serve them.

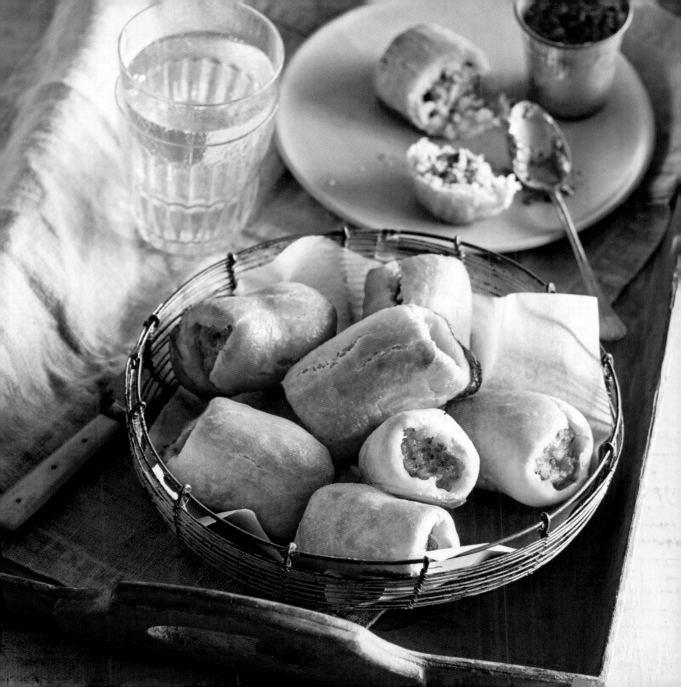

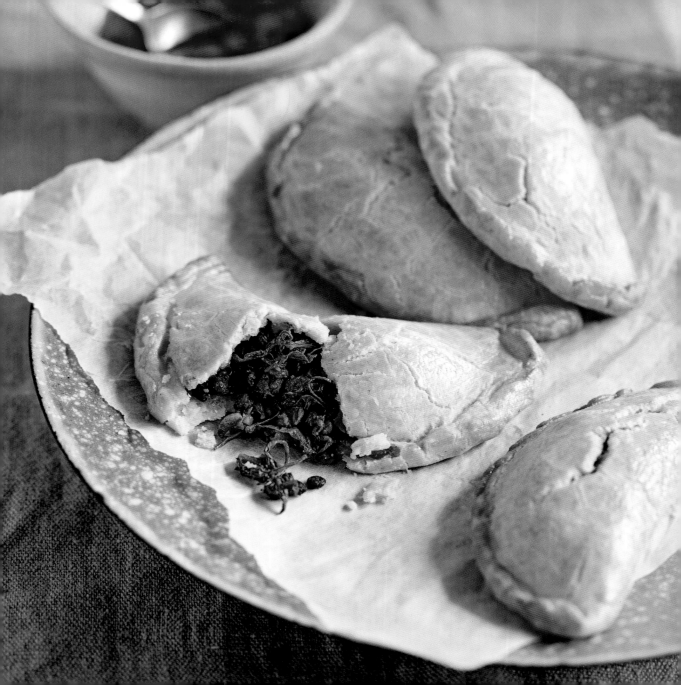

1 tablespoon olive oil

½ red onion, finely chopped

1 garlic clove, finely chopped

1 teaspoon cumin seeds

1 teaspoon dried chilli/hot red pepper flakes

1 teaspoon garam masala

1 teapoon sea salt

200 g/1 cup Puy lentils, cooked

200 g/7 oz. spinach

1 egg, beaten

for the hot water pastry

290 g/2 cups plain/all-purpose gluten-free flour, plus extra for dusting

½ teaspoon xanthan gum

½ teaspoon sea salt

100 g/7 tablespoons vegetable shortening, cubed

1 egg

125 g/½ cup water, recently boiled

a baking sheet lined with non-stick baking parchment or a silicone baking sheet

makes 5–6

These pasties are delicious and you can adapt the filling, adding cheese or mushrooms, or shredded roast chicken if you prefer. They are quite delicate – take care to avoid the pastry breaking.

lentil & spinach pasties

To make the hot water pastry, put the dry ingredients and cubed vegetable shortening into a food processor and pulse to fine crumbs. Pour in the egg, mix briefly and then, with the processor still running, slowly pour in the hot water and mix until completely combined – the mixture will be smooth and almost paste-like. Use a metal spoon to scrape the mixture onto a piece of lightly floured clingfilm/plastic wrap. Wrap the pastry in the clingfilm/plastic wrap and shape into a disc. Chill in the fridge for at least 3 hours.

To make the filling, heat the oil in a saucepan and sauté the onion and garlic until the onion is soft. Add the spices and salt, stir and cook for 2 minutes more. Stir in the lentils and remove from the heat. In another saucepan, wilt the spinach with a teaspoon of water. Drain, pushing the spinach onto a fine-mesh sieve/strainer to remove the excess liquid. Chop the spinach and stir into the lentils, and set aside to cool.

Preheat the oven to 190°C (375°F) Gas 5. Take the pastry from the fridge and break off a 100-g/3½-oz. piece, weighing it out. Roll into a ball with your hands. Lay a piece of clingfilm/plastic wrap onto the work surface. Place the pastry piece in the middle and lay a second piece of clingfilm/plastic wrap on top. Roll out the pastry to a circle of 4–5 mm/ ¼ inch thick. Remove the top layer of clingfilm/plastic wrap and place two tablespoons of the filling mixture into the middle of one side of the pastry disc. Using the clingfilm/plastic wrap to help you, pull one side of the disc over the filling so that it meets the other side, forming a crescent shape. Press down the edges to seal and trim away the excess. Crimp the edges lightly using a fork and then transfer to the lined baking sheet.

Repeat with the remaining pastry and filling, and once all the pasties are ready, brush the tops with the beaten egg. Bake in the preheated oven for 15–20 minutes until golden. Remove, let cool for a few minutes and serve.

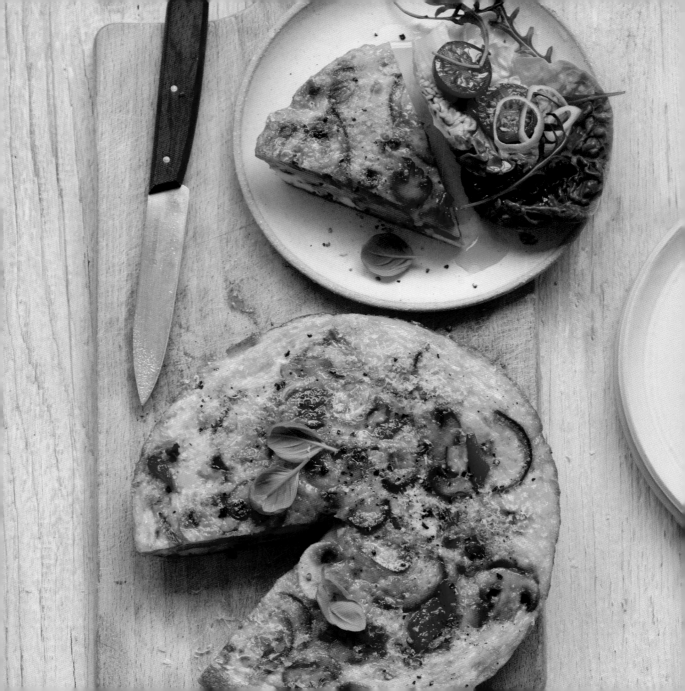

light meals

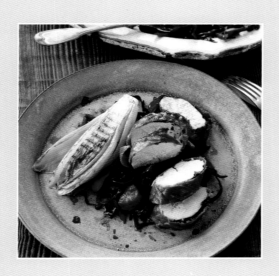

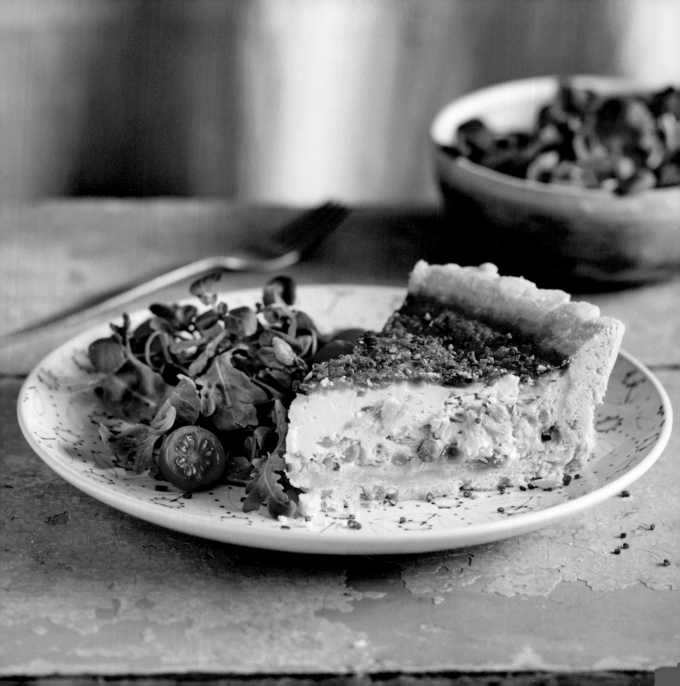

salmon & pea quiche

You can vary the filling in this great staple bake, just keep the egg and cream mixture constant and try combinations of feta and black olive, Cheddar cheese and bacon, or spinach and asparagus.

5 eggs

500 ml/2 cups double/heavy cream

1 teaspoon freshly ground black pepper

2 teaspoons sea salt

2 tablespoons snipped fresh chives, plus extra to serve

125 g/1 cup frozen peas

125 g/4½ oz. smoked salmon, chopped

simple mixed leaf and tomato salad, to serve (optional)

for the shortcrust pastry

460 g/3 cups plain/all-purpose gluten-free flour, plus extra for dusting

1 teaspoon xanthan gum

1 teaspoon sea salt

225 g/15 tablespoons unsalted butter, cubed

1 egg

a 23-cm/9-inch round deep quiche pan, greased

serves 6–8

To make the pastry, put the dry ingredients and cubed butter into a food processor and pulse until they reach a fine crumb consistency. Pour in the egg and 1–2 teaspoons of water and mix until completely combined; the mixture will start to come together. Remove from the bowl and bring together the dough. Lightly knead into a ball and put onto a piece of clingfilm/plastic wrap, press into a disc shape and chill in the fridge for at least 2 hours, until firm. Bring the pastry back to room temperature.

Preheat the oven to 190°C (375°F) Gas 5. Lay a large piece of clingfilm/plastic wrap onto the work surface and lightly dust with flour. Place the pastry in the middle of the clingfilm/plastic wrap, lay a second piece of clingfilm/plastic wrap over the top and roll out the pastry to a 40–45 cm/16–18 inch-diameter circle with a thickness of 5 mm/¼ inch. Gently lift and press the pastry into the pan, and trim the excess pastry away.

Line the case with a piece of baking parchment, then cover with baking beans. Transfer to a baking sheet and blind bake in the preheated oven for 20 minutes. Remove the beans and parchment, then return the case to the oven to bake for another 5–10 minutes until golden. Remove from the oven and set aside. Reduce the heat to 120°C (250°F) Gas ½.

In a jug/pitcher, whisk together the eggs, cream, pepper, salt and chives. Spread half of the frozen peas over the base of the quiche case, along with half of the smoked salmon. Pour the egg mixture into the pastry case and then sprinkle over the remaining peas and salmon. Return the quiche, still on its baking sheet, to the oven and bake for 1–1½ hours until the filling is almost set but has a slight wobble to the centre.

Remove from the oven and cool in the pan on a wire rack for an hour. Refrigerate for at least 2 hours before carefully removing from the pan and slicing into generous wedges (it will be much easier to cut when it is more firmly set). Gently warm if you wish and serve sprinkled with chives.

bean, lemon & herb potato cakes

350 g/12 oz. Jersey Royals or Cornish new potatoes, halved

150 g/1 cup fresh broad/fava beans, shelled

grated zest of 2 lemons

2 tablespoons freshly chopped mint

1 teaspoon ground coriander

150 g/¾ cup natural/plain yogurt

sea salt and freshly ground black pepper

vegetable oil, for shallow frying

serves 4

These delicious potato cakes are ideal for summer entertaining.

Cook the potatoes in a pan of boiling water for 10–15 minutes until tender, drain and cool. Meanwhile cook the beans in a separate pan of boiling water until just tender, drain and cool. Place the beans in a food processor and blend to a coarse paste.

Crush the potatoes and stir in the bean paste, lemon zest, half the mint, the coriander, 1 tablespoon of the yogurt and some seasoning. Divide the mixture into four and use your hands to shape into cakes.

Heat some oil in a large, non-stick frying pan/skillet and fry the cakes for 3 minutes on each side until golden. Mix the remaining yogurt and mint together and serve with the potato cakes.

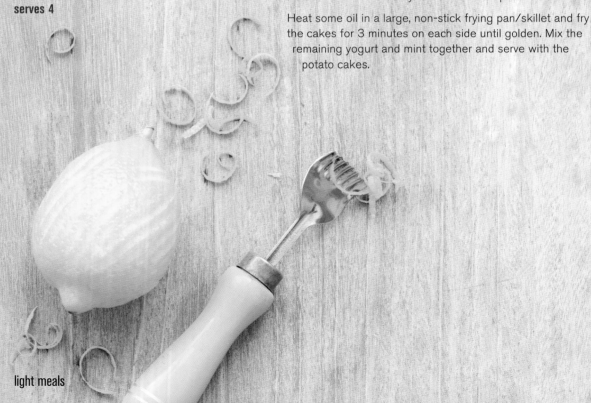

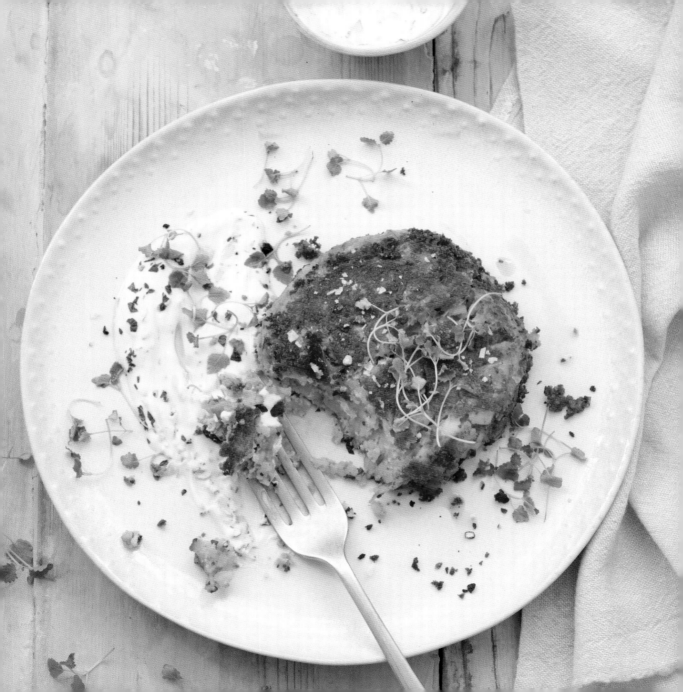

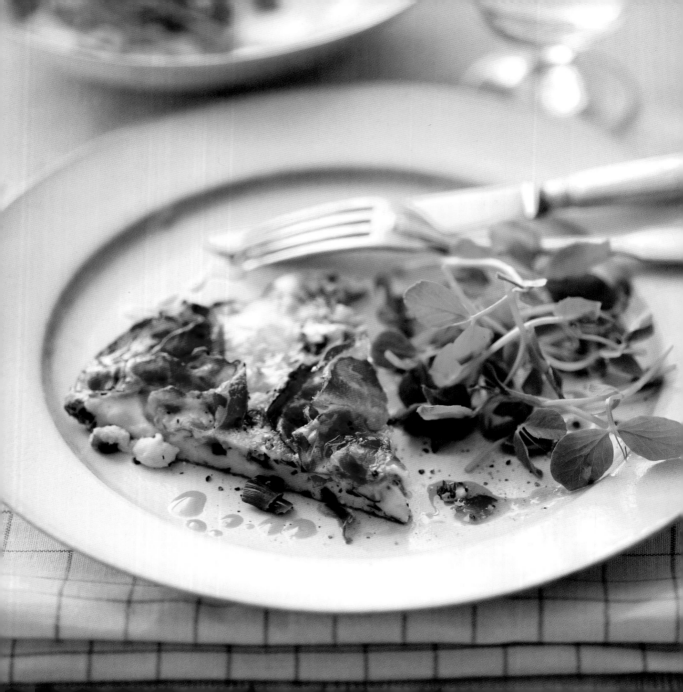

A frittata – the Italian version of an omelette – is an excellent simple meal, and it can also be made as a quiche if you use the shortcrust pastry recipe from the quiche on page 71. Serve with a Pinot Grigio to balance the richness of the cheese and meat.

20 g/generous 1 tablespoon butter

8–10 spring onions/scallions, sliced

6 eggs, beaten

2 tablespoons milk

a big pinch of freshly chopped parsley

1 tablespoon crème fraîche

60 g/2¼ oz. soft goats' cheese (or soft cheese of your choice)

100 g/3¾ oz. coppa or salami, sliced

salt and freshly ground black pepper

salad leaves/greens, to serve

4 lemon quarters, to serve (optional)

serves 4

sliced coppa & spring onion frittata

Heat the butter in a frying pan/skillet until melted, then fry the spring onions/scallions over a high heat, until soft and browned. Meanwhile, mix the eggs with the milk, parsley and some salt and pepper. Pour the beaten egg mixture over the spring onions/scallions and stir once to mix well. Turn the heat down to medium and leave the egg mixture to cook (without stirring) until it starts to thicken.

Meanwhile, preheat the grill/broiler to high.

Once the bottom of the frittata starts to set in the pan, put the crème fraîche on the top of the frittata in evenly spaced 'dollops'. Do the same with pieces of goats' cheese and then with the slices of coppa or salami, pushing the middle of the slices down slightly so that their sides fold up.

Transfer the frying pan/skillet to the preheated grill/broiler and grill/broil for about 5 minutes, until the top browns. Keep checking the frittata regularly to make sure it doesn't burn.

Serve immediately, sliced into wedges. Serve with a side of dressed salad leaves/greens and a lemon quarter to squeeze over the top, if you like.

2 tablespoons olive oil

½ red onion, chopped

½ red (bell) pepper, deseeded and cut into short 1-cm/½-inch-thick strips

150 g/5 oz. white/cup mushrooms, halved

50 g/3 artichokes in oil, well-drained and chopped

4 sun-dried tomatoes in oil, chopped

6 eggs

2 tablespoons grated Parmesan cheese

a handful of fresh basil leaves, roughly torn

2 tablespoons butter

sea salt and freshly ground black pepper

a 25-cm/10-inch heavy-based frying pan/skillet

serves 4

A frittata can be served freshly made or at room temperature. A mixture of mushrooms, onions, sun-dried tomatoes and artichokes gives body and flavour to this savoury egg dish. Serve it with a fresh salad on the side for a light lunch or supper.

tricolore mushroom frittata

Heat the olive oil over a medium heat in a frying pan/skillet. Fry the onion and red (bell) pepper for 3 minutes, until softened. Add the mushrooms and fry for 3 minutes. Remove from the pan; set aside to cool. When cool, mix together with the artichokes and sun-dried tomatoes. Wipe the pan clean.

Thoroughly whisk the eggs together in a mixing bowl. Season with salt and freshly ground black pepper. Mix in the Parmesan, the cooled vegetable mixture and the basil leaves.

Heat the butter in the frying pan/skillet over a medium heat, until frothing. Add the egg mixture, spreading it to form an even layer. Reduce the heat to low and cook for 15–20 minutes, until the base of the frittata has set, but the surface is still liquid.

Preheat the grill/broiler to high. Place the frittata under the grill/broiler for 1–2 minutes until the surface has set. Serve warm or at room temperature, cut into wedges.

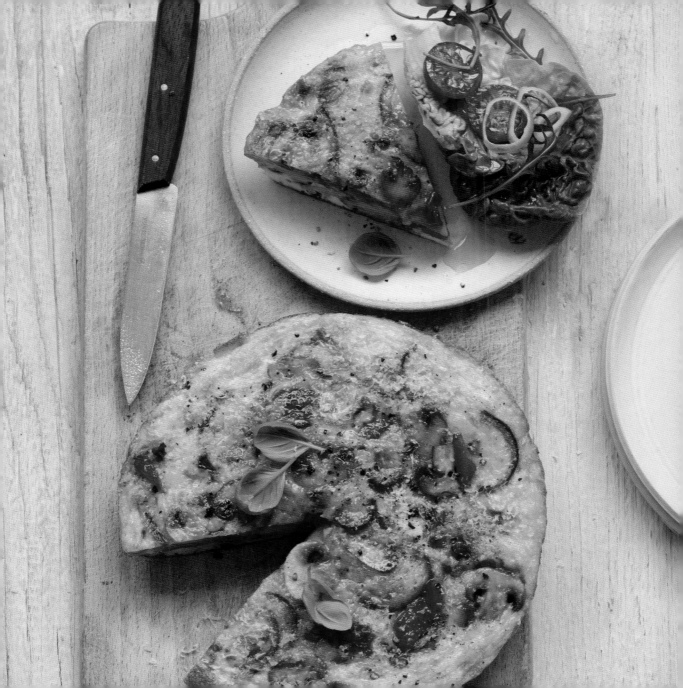

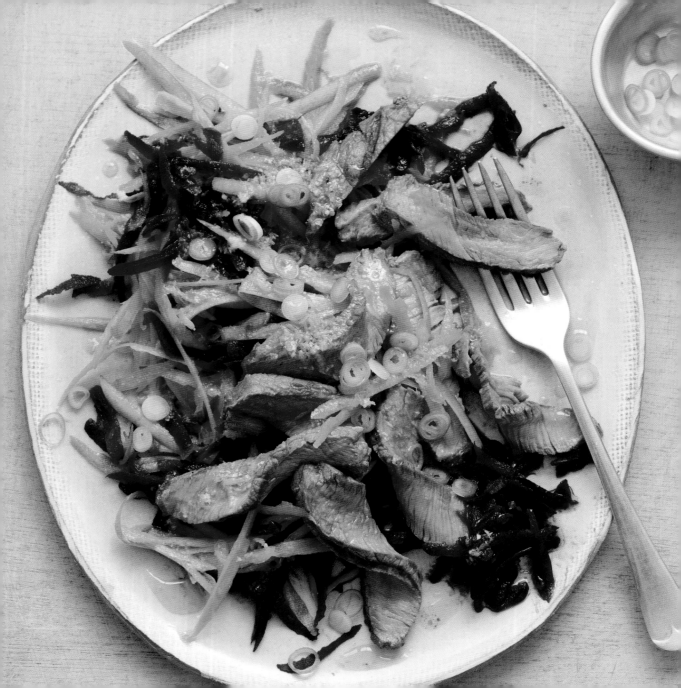

seared beef salad

4 medium beetroot/beets

400 g/14 oz. sirloin steak

2 tablespoons olive oil

1 tablespoon horseradish sauce

grated zest and freshly squeezed juice of 2 lemons

2 spring onions/scallions, trimmed and sliced

4 carrots, peeled and coarsely grated

1 tablespoon good-quality balsamic vinegar

sea salt and freshly ground black pepper

a ridged stove-top griddle/grill pan

serves 4

This salad has a hint of an oriental feel and will taste all the better if you use the very best steaks that you can find.

Place the beetroot/beets in a large pan of water, bring to the boil, reduce the heat and simmer for 30 minutes. Drain the beetroot/beets and set aside to cool. Once cool, carefully peel off the skin and coarsely grate.

Season the sirloin steak with salt and pepper and brush with the olive oil. Heat the griddle until hot and sauté the steak, 3–4 minutes on each side for rare, 8–10 minutes for medium, turning once.

In a large bowl combine the beetroot/beets, horseradish, lemon zest and juice, spring onions/scallions, carrots and balsamic vinegar. Slice the beef and serve on top of the salad.

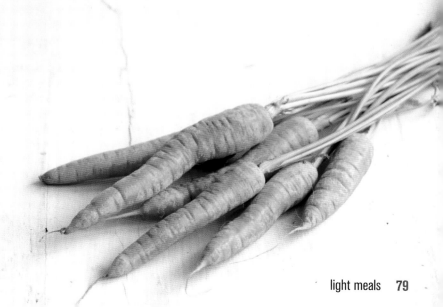

salmon escabeche with celery & citrus

2 tablespoons olive oil

4 boneless salmon fillets, skinned

2 shallots, sliced into thin rounds

2 fennel bulbs, trimmed and thinly sliced, reserve the fronds to garnish

4 celery stalks, as white as possible, thinly sliced

3 fresh bay leaves

4 garlic cloves, thinly sliced

grated zest of 2 lemons and freshly squeezed juice of 1

grated zest of 2 limes and freshly squeezed juice of 1

a handful of fresh mint leaves

sea salt and freshly ground black pepper

serves 4

Fennel, celery and fish are a marriage made in heaven. Here, the fish is prepared the Spanish way: escabeche is a method of searing fish or meat and then marinating it in a tangy citrus dressing. Do try it with other fish – mackerel is divine.

Heat the oil in a large, non-stick frying pan/skillet. Season the salmon fillets with salt and fry over a medium heat for 3 minutes on each side until a little opaque. Set aside to rest.

Return the pan to the heat. Add the shallots, fennel, celery and bay leaves. Season and cook for 5 minutes. Add the garlic and cook for a further 2 minutes. Remove from the heat. Now add the citrus zest and juice along with 4 tablespoons of water.

Add the fish to this citrus mixture and spoon the juices over to coat the fish. Arrange on a platter with the mint leaves and fennel fronds, and serve with crusty gluten-free bread to mop up the juices.

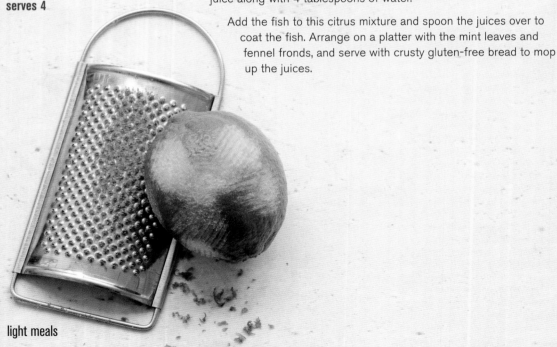

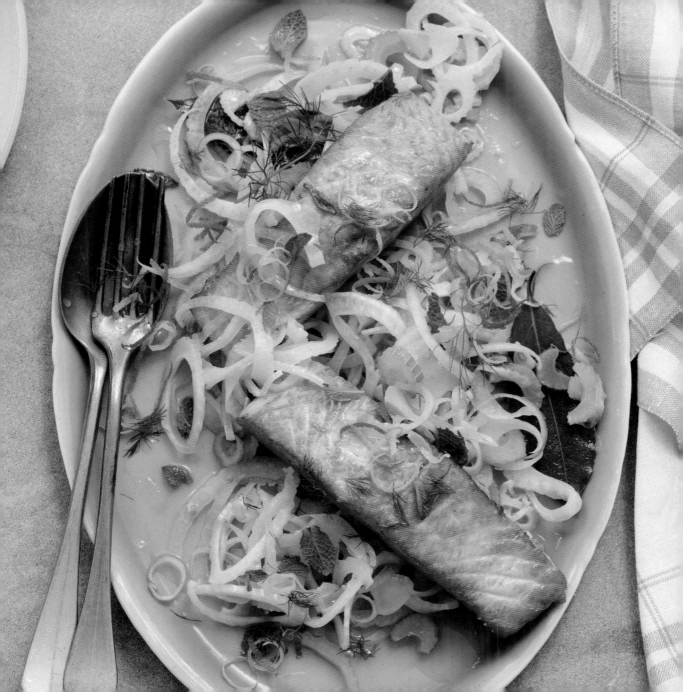

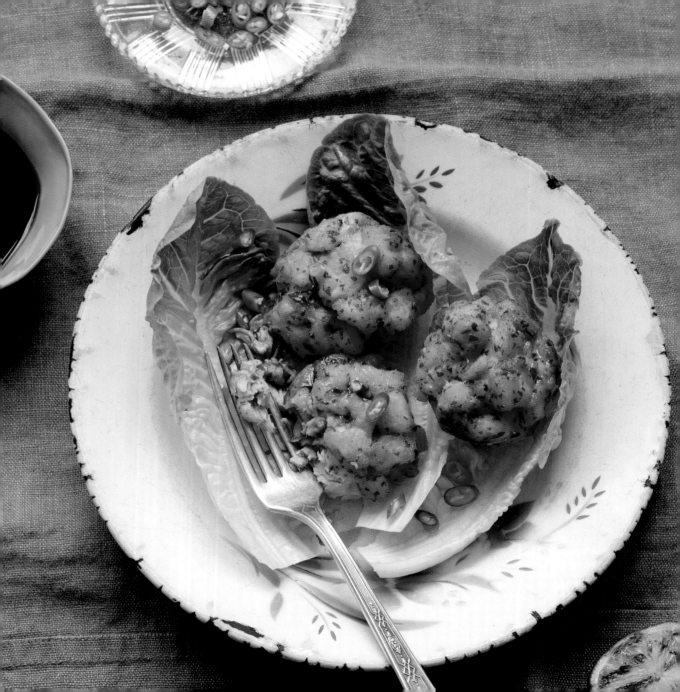

500 g/1¼ lb. salmon fillets, skin removed

1 egg white

3 tablespoons fine rice flour

2 fresh kaffir lime leaves, shredded

1 tablespoon peeled and finely chopped fresh ginger

1 teaspoon wasabi paste

3 tablespoons freshly chopped flat-leaf parsley leaves

vegetable oil, for shallow frying

Little Gem/Bibb lettuce leaves, to serve (optional)

sliced green and red chillies/chiles, to garnish

for the lime dipping sauce

freshly squeezed juice of 2 limes

4 tablespoons gluten-free soy sauce

2 tablespoons brown sugar

makes 20

An indispensable part of authentic Thai cooking, kaffir lime leaves are used to give a sharply aromatic edge to many dishes. These fish cakes make a wonderful appetizer or even light lunch served with the dipping sauce and rice and salad on the side.

salmon & kaffir lime cakes

Remove any bones from the salmon and finely dice into small cubes. In a large bowl, combine the diced salmon with the egg white, rice flour, kaffir lime leaves, ginger, wasabi and parsley. Mix together until well combined.

Preheat the oven to 120°C (250°F) Gas ½.

Pour in enough oil to coat the base of a frying pan/skillet and set over a medium heat. Put 2 tablespoons of salmon mixture per cake into the hot oil and cook for 35–45 seconds on each side until lightly golden. Depending on the size of your pan, you can cook these in batches of around six at a time. Drain on paper towels, then transfer to a non-stick baking sheet and keep warm in the oven while you cook the rest.

To make the dipping sauce, simply mix together the ingredients in a small dish. Serve the warm fish cakes in lettuce leaves, if liked, and sprinkled with sliced chillies/chiles, with the dipping sauce on the side.

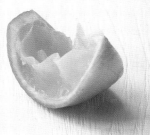

Although a humble staple, cauliflower is deservedly beginning to garner attention from foodies. This velvety purée is so good it could even, blitzed with cooking water, stand alone as a soup.

sea bass, cauliflower purée & Swiss chard

extra virgin olive oil

1 onion, diced

4 garlic cloves, crushed

1 head of cauliflower, cut into florets, (about 450 g/1 lb.)

vegetable stock, about 800 ml/scant 3½ cups or enough to cover

1 bunch Swiss chard, about 400 g/ 14 oz., leaves removed from the thick stalks, both reserved

4 sea bass fillets, skin on

small bunch of fresh flat-leaf parsley, finely chopped

sea salt and freshly ground black pepper

parsley oil, to serve

serves 4

Pour 2 tablespoons of olive oil into a large frying pan/skillet over a medium heat. Add the onion and sweat for 10 minutes until soft. Add almost all of the garlic and cook for 1 minute, then add the cauliflower, stir everything together and cook for 2 minutes.

Pour in enough vegetable stock to barely cover the cauliflower. Bring to the boil, reduce the heat and simmer until very soft. Drain off the stock through a sieve/strainer and discard. Put the cooked onion, garlic and cauliflower into a food processor. Blitz until you have a very smooth purée, adding in a drizzle of olive oil, if needed. Taste and adjust the seasoning, if necessary. Keep the mixture warm.

Place the chard stalks in a large pot of boiling salted water. Cook until just tender, but not limp. This should take about 3–4 minutes, depending on the thickness of the chard – taste a small piece to check. Remove, drain and season with a pinch of salt and a drizzle of olive oil. Boil the chard leaves in the same way, but remove after 2 minutes, drain well and season with salt and olive oil. Keep warm.

Place two non-stick frying pans/skillets over a medium-high heat. Drizzle a little olive oil over the sea bass fillets, just enough to coat both sides. Season with salt and pepper and when hot, place two fillets in each pan, skin-side down. Fry for 3 minutes without moving, then turn over and fry for a further 2 minutes.

Mix the chopped parsley and remaining crushed garlic with a pinch of salt and enough olive oil to create a loose parsley oil.

Spoon some of the cauliflower purée onto each plate, place a sea bass fillet on top with the chard twisted in and around the fish. Drizzle over some parsley oil and serve.

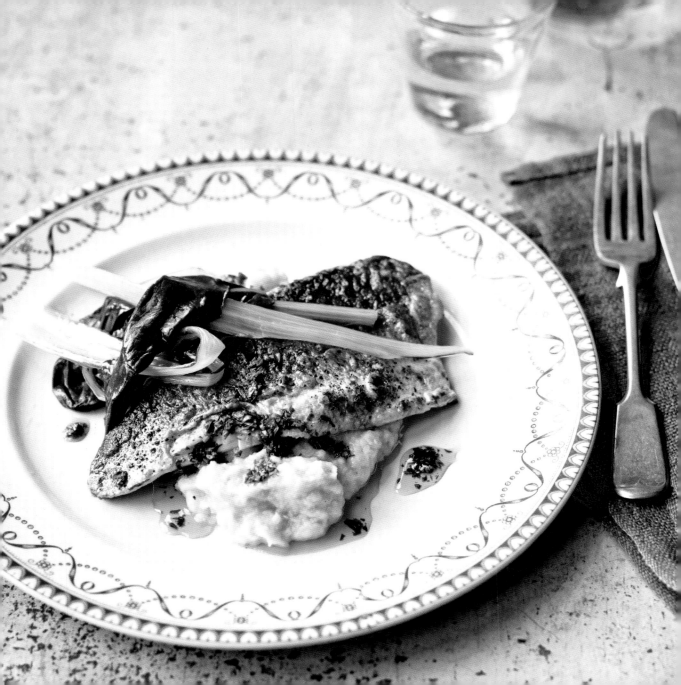

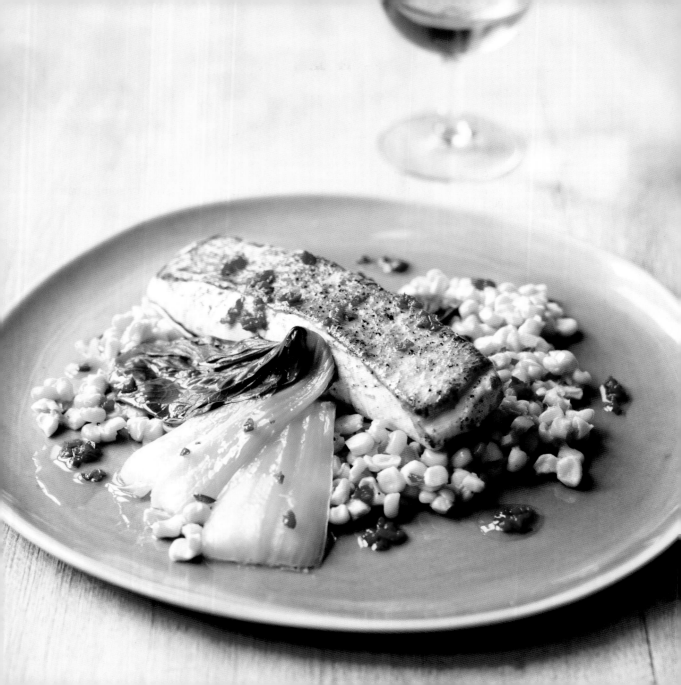

halibut & coconut creamed corn with pak choi & chilli oil

4 corn on the cob/ears fresh corn

300 ml/1¼ cups coconut cream (thick cream from the top of coconut milk; you can also use coconut milk but it will be a little thinner in consistency)

sea salt

¼ teaspoon paprika

handful of coriander/cilantro leaves

grated zest of 1 lime, plus 1 teaspoon freshly squeezed juice

100 g/3½ oz. pak choi/bok choy

extra virgin olive oil

1 fresh red chilli/chile, halved and deseeded

4 x 150 g/5 oz. halibut fillets, skin on

sea salt and freshly ground black pepper

serves 4

This coconut creamed corn is totally addictive, and works well as a side for most fish dishes, or on its own tossed with some salad for lunch. Try to buy sustainably-caught halibut – look out for the MSC (Marine Stewardship Council) certification, or ask your fishmonger.

Using a serrated knife cut the corn kernels off the cob; the easiest way to do this is to stand the cob upright and cut down in a sawing motion.

Add the corn, coconut cream and 1 teaspoon of salt to a frying pan/skillet and set over a medium-high heat. Bring to the boil, then reduce the heat to low and simmer for about 20 minutes until the corn is tender and the coconut cream has reduced. Add in the paprika, coriander/cilantro, lime zest and juice and season with black pepper.

While the corn is cooking, bring a saucepan of water to the boil, add in a good pinch of salt and cook the pak choi/bok choy for a couple of minutes until just tender. I like them to still have a bit of bite. Drain and season with a drizzle of olive oil and a little salt. Keep warm.

Chop the chilli/chile very finely, then place in a small bowl with 3 tablespoons of olive oil and a pinch of salt, and set aside.

Place two frying pans/skillets over a medium-high heat. Season the halibut fillets with salt and pepper and drizzle olive oil over both sides of each fillet. Once the pans are hot, place two halibut fillets in each pan, skin-side down. Let them sizzle for about 2–3 minutes, then turn over and cook for another 2–3 minutes (depending on their respective thickness) until they are just cooked through.

To serve, spoon some creamed corn onto a plate, place the halibut on top and twist over the pak choi/bok choy. Drizzle over the chilli oil and serve.

teriyaki salmon

Teriyaki is a delicious sauce, made incredibly simply and it stores for weeks. The word refers to the sugar glaze (teri) and the cooking method of grilling/broiling the meat (yaki), so the idea is to cook the fish in the teriyaki sauce until it has reduced to a tasty, sticky glaze. Only use a medium or low heat as the sauce can catch and burn easily due to the high sugar content. Do not leave it cooking unsupervised. The sauce works well with most fish and is sometimes used for meat too – try pork or chicken.

100 g/generous ½ cup long-grain rice

a pinch of sea salt

4 salmon fillets (each about 120 g/ 4 oz.)

2 tablespoons sesame oil

2 heads of pak choi/bok choy, sliced in half

a 5-cm/2-in. piece of fresh ginger, peeled and finely grated

2 spring onions/scallions, thinly sliced

for the teriyaki sauce

200 ml/¾ cup mirin

50 ml/3½ tablespoons tamari

100 g/½ cup caster/granulated sugar

serves 4

First, make the teriyaki sauce. Put the mirin and tamari with the sugar in a small pan set over a gentle heat. Simmer for 2 minutes and stir until all the ingredients are combined. Remove from the heat and set aside.

Next, cook the rice. Bring 300 ml/1¼ cups of water to the boil in a saucepan set over a medium heat. Add the rice and salt, and bring back to the boil. Once boiling, take the pan off the heat, cover and set aside to allow the rice to cook for 15 minutes.

Meanwhile, to prepare the salmon fillets, carefully remove the skin using a small sharp knife and check the flesh for any bones with your fingertips, removing and discarding any you find with fish tweezers.

Set a non-stick frying pan/skillet over a medium heat and pour in the oil. Heat until the oil just starts to smoke, then carefully place the salmon fillets in the pan. Cook until half of each fillet has coloured before adding the teriyaki sauce to the pan. Cover and simmer for 5 minutes. Carefully spoon over the teriyaki sauce, then remove the salmon to a clean plate using a fish slice. Cover with foil to keep warm.

Turn up the heat and reduce the remaining sauce for 2 minutes, until it has started to thicken. Place the pak choi/bok choy cut-side down in the pan, cover and cook for 1 minute so that it just cooks in the steam.

To serve, strain the cooked rice and place a spoonful in each large bowl. Place some pak choi/bok choy on top, then the salmon. Sprinkle grated ginger over the plate then finish with the sliced spring onions/scallion.

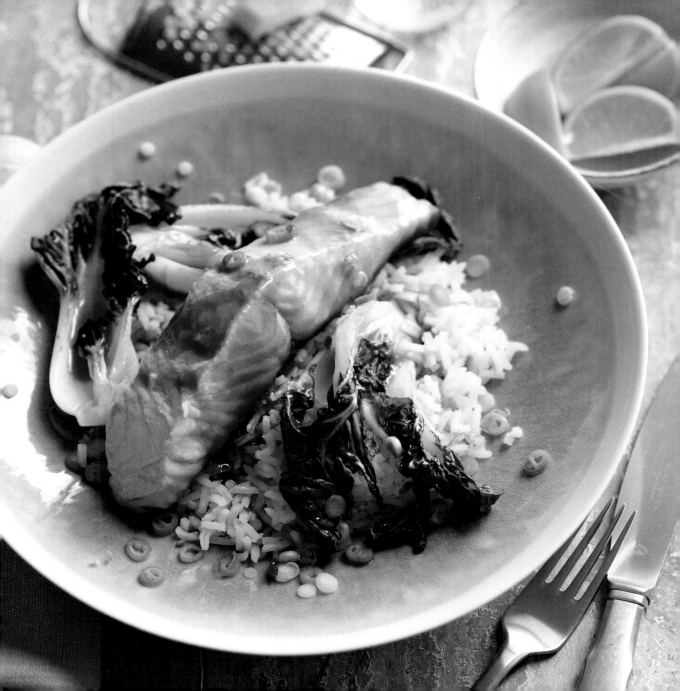

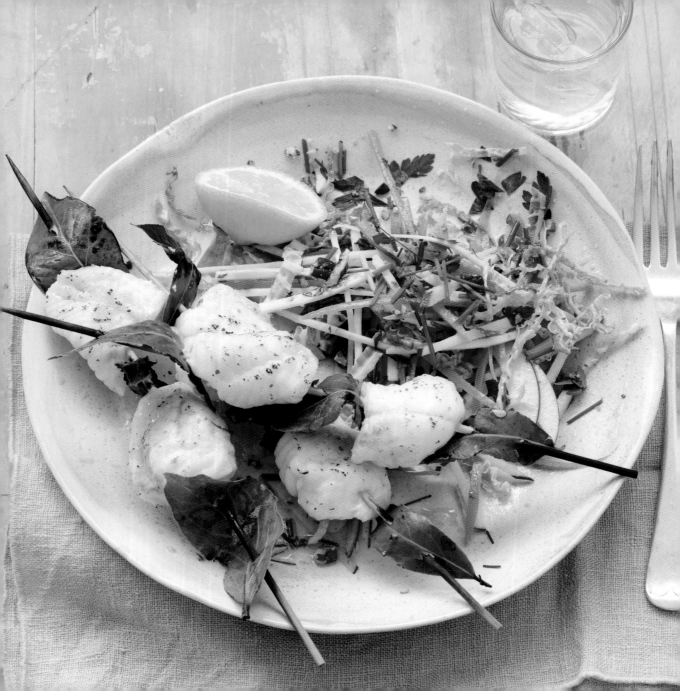

for the vegetable slaw

2 red dessert apples, cored

2 medium carrots, peeled

300 g/2 cups celeriac, peeled and grated

200 g/2 cups savoy cabbage, finely shredded

a handful of fresh flat-leaf parsley, finely chopped

a handful of fresh chives, finely chopped

40 g/⅓ cup pecans, roasted and roughly chopped

5 tablespoons buttermilk

5 tablespoons extra virgin olive oil

grated zest of 1 lemon, plus freshly squeezed juice of ½

sea salt and freshly ground black pepper

for the skewers

1 kg/2¼ lbs. monkfish tails, skinned

36 large fresh bay leaves

olive oil, for brushing

lemon halves or wedges, to serve

12 bamboo barbecue skewers, soaked in cold water

serves 4

Ideal for relaxed entertaining, you can either cook these on the barbecue or under the grill/broiler. Bay leaves, fish and lemon are a flavour match made in heaven. Forge a good relationship with your fishmonger — then they can skin the monkfish for you.

monkfish & bay leaf skewers with lemon & vegetable slaw

To make the vegetable slaw, cut the apples and the carrots into small, slim matchsticks. Place the sliced vegetables in a large bowl with the grated celeriac, shredded cabbage, fresh herbs and chopped pecans.

In a separate bowl combine the buttermilk, olive oil, lemon zest and juice. Season to taste with salt and pepper and stir together. Pour onto the vegetables and toss to mix. Set the slaw aside in the refrigerator until ready to serve.

Cut the monkfish tails into 24 even-sized pieces of around 5 cm/2 in. each. Thread three bay leaves and two pieces of monkfish alternately onto each of the pre-soaked bamboo skewers, starting and ending with a bay leaf. Brush the fish with olive oil and season with salt and pepper.

Preheat a barbecue or grill/broiler to medium. Cook the skewers on/under the heat for 2 minutes on each side until the fish is cooked through. Serve with the slaw and lemon to squeeze over.

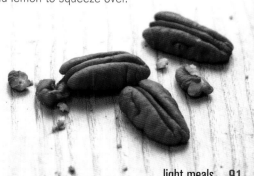

16 white/cup mushrooms, stalks trimmed off

250 g/9 oz. boneless chicken breast, cut into short, thin strips

16 fresh shiitake mushrooms, halved, stalks trimmed off

½ green (bell) pepper, deseeded and cut into 2- x 2-cm/¾- x ¾-inch squares

2 spring onions/scallions, cut into 2-cm/¾-inch lengths

finely chopped red chilli/chile, to garnish (optional)

for the yakitori glaze

50 ml/3½ tablespoons rice wine or Amontillado sherry

50 ml/3½ tablespoons mirin

50 ml/3½ tablespoons tamari

1 tablespoon caster/granulated sugar

¼ teaspoon sea salt

8 metal or bamboo barbecue skewers, soaked in cold water

serves 4

These salty-sweet glazed chicken skewers invariably go down well! Fresh shiitake mushrooms, with their distinctive flavour, are a pleasing element in the dish. Serve with jasmine or sushi rice and blanched pak choi/bok choy, Chinese broccoli or spinach.

yakitori-glazed mushroom & chicken skewers

Make the yakitori glaze by placing the rice wine or sherry, mirin, tamari, sugar and salt in a small saucepan. Bring to the boil and boil for 1 minute until melted together into a syrupy glaze. Turn off the heat.

Thread the white/cup mushrooms, chicken, shiitake mushrooms, green (bell) pepper and spring onions/scallions onto the eight skewers.

Preheat the grill/broiler. Brush the skewers generously with the yakitori glaze. Grill/broil the skewers for 8–10 minutes, until the chicken is cooked through, brushing repeatedly with the glaze and turning the skewers over halfway through. Serve at once, garnished with red chilli/chile, if liked.

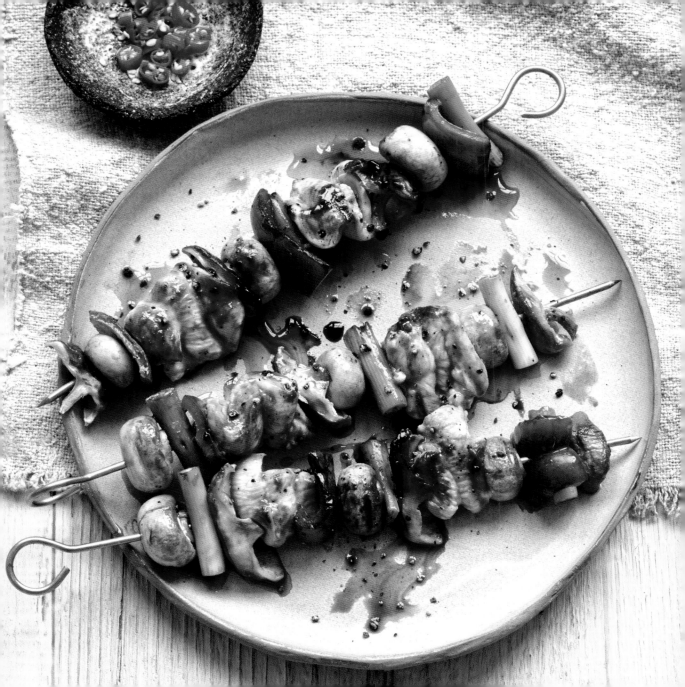

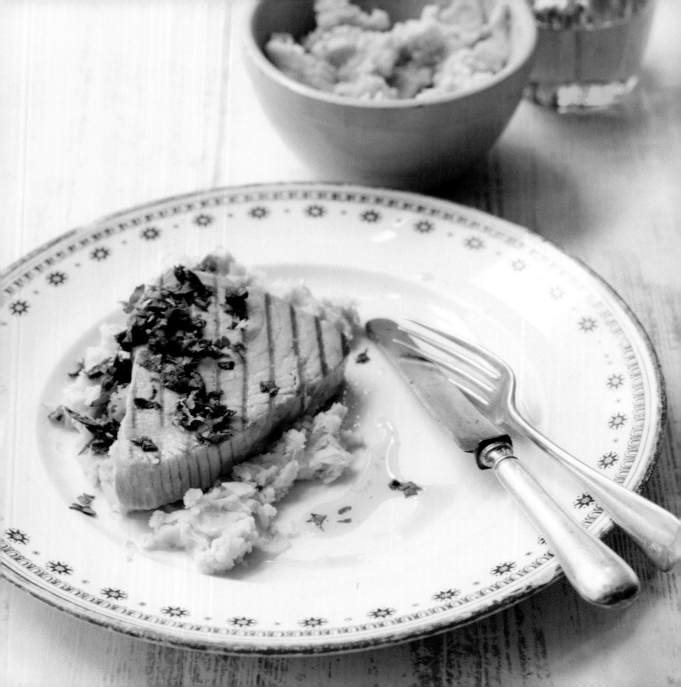

griddled tuna with garlic bean purée & gremolata

2 x 400-g/14-oz. cans of butter/lima beans in water

2 tablespoons olive oil

1 onion, finely chopped

1 garlic clove, finely chopped

4 tuna steaks, each approximately 200 g/7 oz.

sea salt and freshly ground black pepper

extra virgin olive oil, to garnish

for the gremolata

2 garlic cloves, peeled

pinch of sea salt

finely grated zest of 2 lemons

6 tablespoons freshly chopped parsley

a ridged stove-top griddle/grill pan

serves 4

Gremolata – traditionally served with osso buco – also goes very well with fish. Here, firm-textured tuna steaks contrast nicely with the soft bean purée, while gremolata adds a refreshing zip. A great dish to make for dinner parties.

First, make the gremolata. Crush the garlic cloves with a pinch of salt to a paste. Mix together with the lemon zest and parsley and set aside.

Drain the beans, reserving 4 tablespoons of the bean water. Heat 1 tablespoon of the olive oil in a heavy-bottomed saucepan. Add the onion and garlic and fry gently, stirring, until softened. Add the drained butter/lima beans and reserved bean water, mixing in. Cover and cook gently for 10 minutes, stirring now and then. Mash into a purée, season with salt and pepper and keep warm until serving.

Preheat the griddle/grill pan until very hot. Brush the tuna steaks with the remaining olive oil and season with salt and pepper. Griddle the tuna steaks until cooked to taste (about 2–3 minutes per side), turning occasionally to ensure even cooking.

Spoon the gremolata over the griddled tuna steaks and serve on a bed of bean purée, drizzling over a little extra virgin olive oil for flavour and moisture.

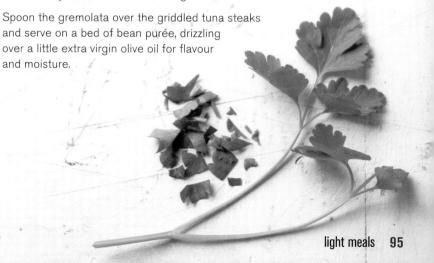

mackerel kedgeree

1 brown onion, diced

2 teaspoons garam masala

1 teaspoon ground turmeric

200 g/1½ cups long-grain rice

a pinch of sea salt

4 hard-boiled/hard-cooked eggs

50 g/⅓ cup frozen peas

2 red chillies/chiles, thinly sliced

a small bunch of fresh flat-leaf parsley

2 smoked mackerel fillets, skinned and flaked

50 ml/3½ tablespoons double/heavy cream

vegetable oil, for frying

serves 4

Originating in India as a breakfast dish called 'khichdi', kedgeree (a fish and curried rice dish) was brought back to the United Kingdom in Victorian times and modified as part of the Anglo-Indian cuisine of the time. There are few better morning-after meals to be had. Although traditionally cooked with smoked haddock, do try it with any smoked fish; here it is made with smoked mackerel. Use a good-quality garam masala.

Add just enough oil to cover the base of a medium saucepan and set over a medium heat. Add the onion, garam masala and turmeric and heat for a couple of minutes before adding the rice. Stir to coat the rice in oil and spice, then add 400 ml/1⅔ cups of water and the salt. Bring to a simmer, then take the pan off the heat, cover and set aside to allow the rice to cook for 15 minutes.

Peel and quarter the boiled eggs and set aside.

Once the rice is cooked, return to a gentle heat and stir in the frozen peas. Add the chillies/chiles and parsley, reserving some for garnishing, before finally adding the flaked mackerel and cream. Carefully stir all of the ingredients together until evenly mixed and hot.

Transfer the kedgeree to a large serving dish, garnish with the egg quarters and a sprinkling of parsley and serve at the table.

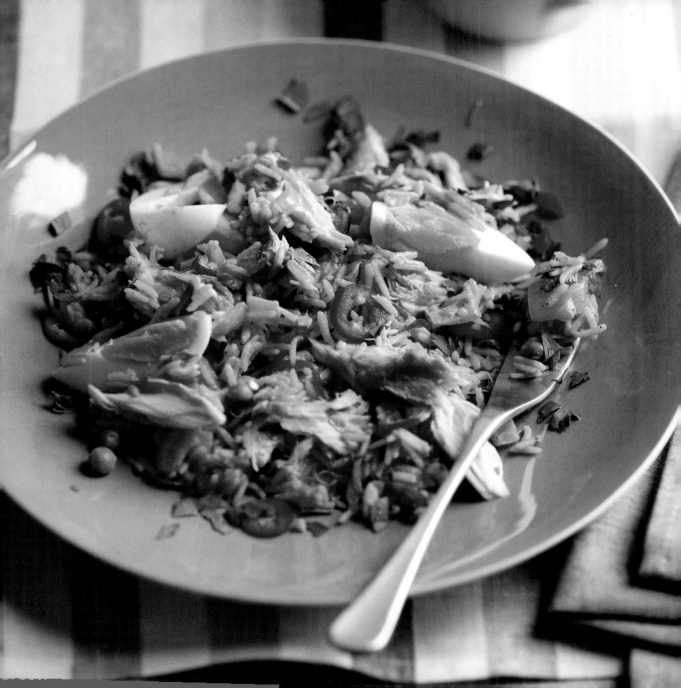

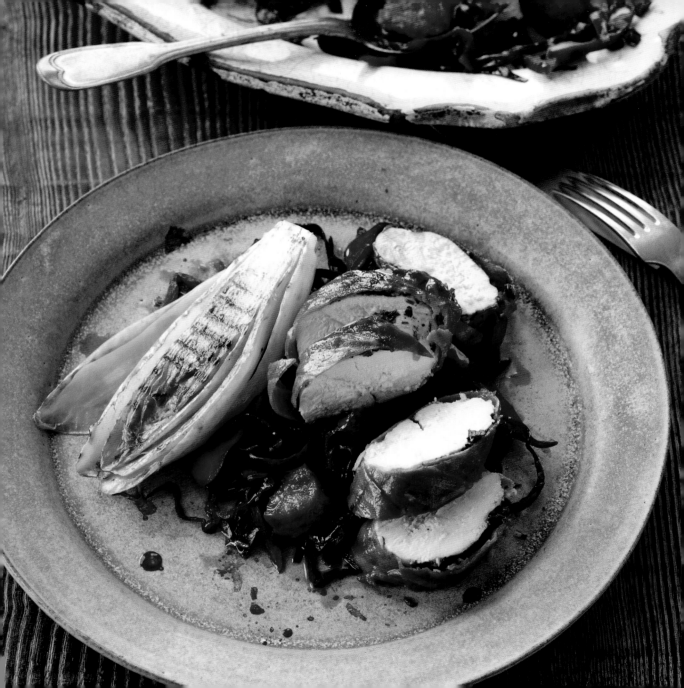

1 tablespoon red wine vinegar

1 tablespoon olive oil, plus extra for griddling

1 teaspoon soft/packed brown sugar

1 garlic clove, finely chopped

a big pinch of freshly chopped parsley

a pinch each of sea salt and freshly ground black pepper

2 skinless, boneless chicken breasts

4 slices prosciutto

1 chicory/Belgian endive, halved

1 teaspoon paprika

for the red cabbage & chorizo salad

1 tablespoon olive oil

½ red cabbage, cored and shredded

150 g/5 oz. gluten-free chorizo, skinned and diced

for the salad dressing

3 tablespoons olive oil

1 tablespoon red wine vinegar

½ teaspoon crushed garlic

a big pinch of freshly chopped parsley

a pinch of freshly chopped or dried tarragon

1 teaspoon freshly squeezed lime juice

a ridged stove-top griddle/grill pan

serves 2

This makes an impressive dinner party dish and works brilliantly served with the red cabbage and chorizo salad.

chicken breasts wrapped in prosciutto with griddled chicory

Put the vinegar, olive oil, sugar, garlic, parsley and salt and pepper in a bowl and mix together, then rub this mixture into the chicken breasts. Wrap the chicken in clingfilm/plastic wrap and leave in the refrigerator for at least 1 hour.

Meanwhile, make the salad. Heat the olive oil in a frying pan/skillet over a medium heat, then add the red cabbage and fry until soft, stirring regularly. Add the chorizo and keep stirring for 2–3 minutes, so that the chorizo starts to cook and releases its oils. Remove from the heat and leave to cool. Put all the dressing ingredients into a bowl and mix well.

Remove the chicken from the refrigerator, then wrap each chicken breast in two 2 slices of prosciutto.

Heat the griddle/grill pan over a high heat with a drop more olive oil added to the pan, then add the prosciutto-wrapped chicken breasts to the hot pan and cook for 6–7 minutes. Place the chicory/Belgian endive halves, flat-sides down, next to the chicken in the same pan. Turn the wrapped breasts and cook on the other side, until cooked through. Sprinkle the paprika over the top of the wrapped breasts and the chicory/Belgian endive.

Turn the wrapped breasts again; you should have the nice brown griddle lines across the prosciutto. Turn the chicory/Belgian endive halves over near the end of cooking time, just to soften the outside, but they're fine face-down for most of the cooking time to get the nice crunchy griddle lines across them. Once the cabbage and chorizo mixture for the salad has cooled, pour over the dressing, toss to mix, and serve with the cooked wrapped breasts and chicory/Belgian endive.

150 g/¾ cup basmati rice

75 g/⅓ cup tandoori paste

75 g/¼ cup natural/plain Greek yogurt

1 tablespoon freshly squeezed lemon juice

1 tablespoon grated zest from lemon

12 French-trimmed lamb cutlets (approximately 600 g/1 lb. 5 oz.)

sea salt and freshly ground black pepper

for the tomato and coriander/ cilantro salsa

200 g/1⅓ cups cherry tomatoes, halved

1 small red onion, finely chopped

grated zest of 1 lemon

2 tablespoons freshly chopped coriander/cilantro leaves

serves 4

Tandoori is northern Indian and relies on spices and yogurt. Colourful and straightforward, this dish is ideal for relaxed entertaining. Serve with poppadoms and lime pickle.

tandoori lamb cutlets with tomato & coriander salsa

Cook the rice according to the packet instructions, then drain.

Meanwhile, preheat the grill/broiler or barbecue to high.

Combine the tandoori paste, yogurt, lemon juice and zest in a large bowl. Add the lamb cutlets and turn to coat the lamb in the mixture. Season.

Cook the lamb under/on the hot grill/broiler or barbecue for 4 minutes each side, or until browned and cooked as desired. Remove from the heat and allow to stand for 5 minutes.

Meanwhile, to make the tomato and coriander/cilantro salsa, combine all the ingredients in a bowl and season to taste with salt and pepper.

Serve the lamb cutlets with the rice and salsa.

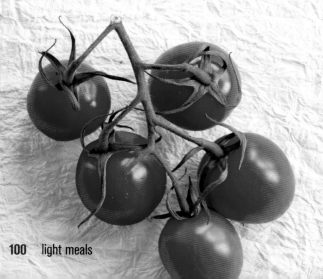

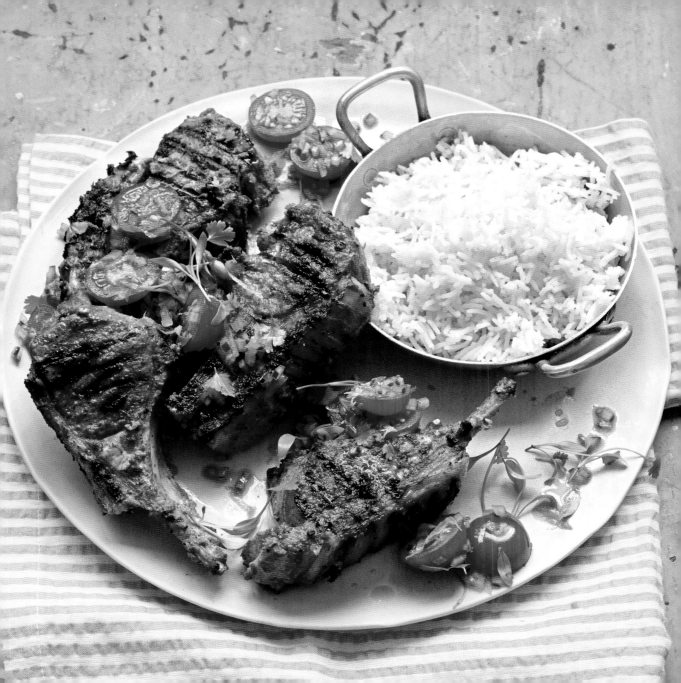

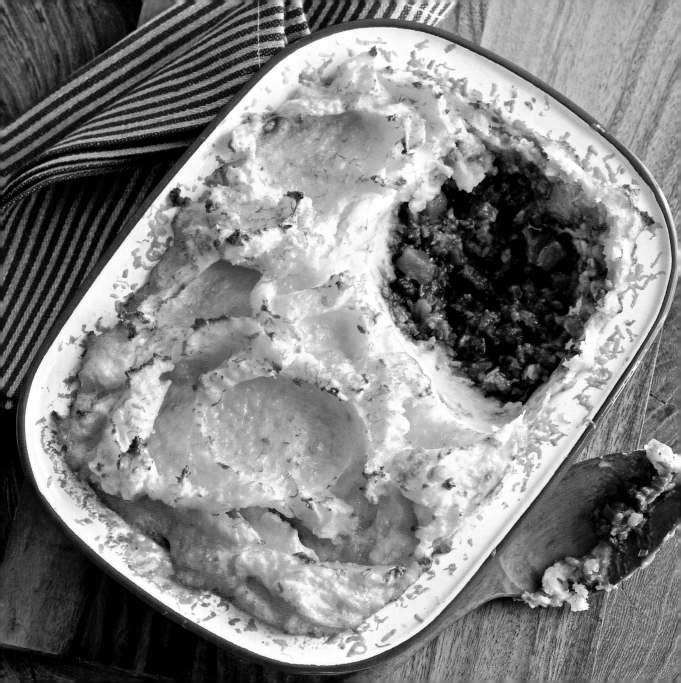

comfort food

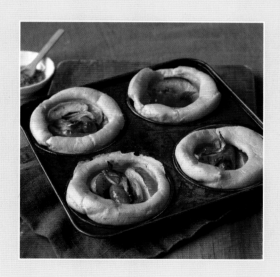

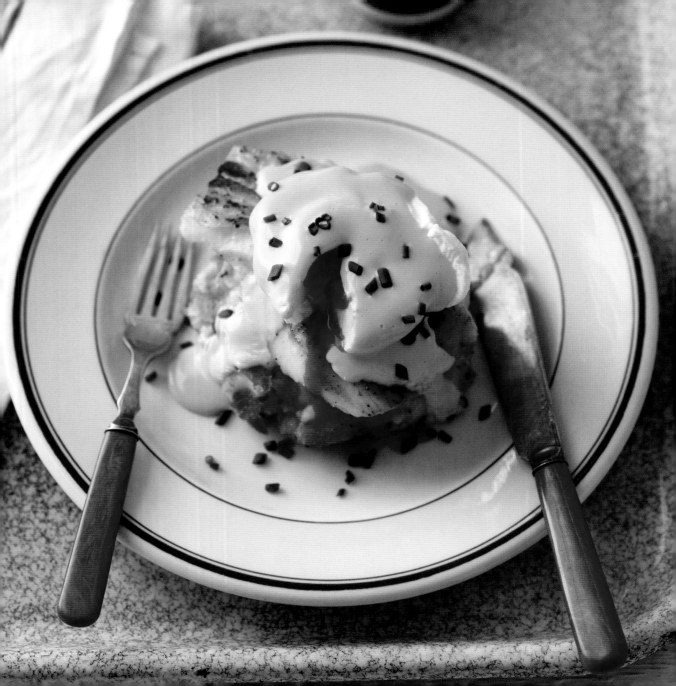

It doesn't get much more comforting than this: a delicious fillet of haddock, an oozy poached egg with hollandaise and fried mashed potato cakes to mop it all up with – heaven on a plate.

haddock with potato cakes, poached egg & hollandaise sauce

600 g/3 cups mashed potatoes

1 teaspoon white wine vinegar

4 eggs

4 x 150 g/5½ oz. haddock fillets, skinned and boned

a small bunch of fresh chives, thinly sliced

sea salt and freshly ground black pepper

butter, for frying

for the hollandaise

250 g/2 sticks plus 1 tablespoon butter

4 egg yolks

a pinch of sea salt

freshly squeezed juice of ½ lemon

a 500-ml/18-oz. capacity jug/pitcher

serves 4

Make the mashed potatoes following your usual method. Set a large frying pan/skillet over a high heat and add a little butter – it should colour and caramelize a little as you cook. Make four patties with the mashed potatoes and put them in the warm pan to cook for 2 minutes on each side. Keep warm in a low oven until ready to serve.

Make the hollandaise just before you start cooking the fish and eggs so it is still hot. Heat the butter in a saucepan set over a low heat until just melted, then leave to cool for a few minutes. Add the egg yolks, a pinch of salt and the lemon juice to the jug/pitcher and whisk on high with a hand-held electric blender. Slowly pour the hot butter, while still whisking, into the jug/pitcher to form a pale yellow sauce.

Bring a large pan of water (about 5-cm/2-in. deep) to the boil over a high heat, add the vinegar and turn off the heat. Break the eggs into the water one at a time and leave to cook in the warm water for 6–8 minutes – you might need to heat the water a little to finish cooking.

Put a knob of butter in a large non-stick frying pan/skillet set over a medium heat until the base is covered and the butter is just starting to foam. Season with salt and place the haddock fillets in the pan. Cook until they are opaque two-thirds of the way through, then finish cooking by spooning over the hot butter – they should be caramelized and brown on the bottom and pale, but cooked on the top.

Serve on large, hot plates. Place a warm potato cake on each plate, then a haddock fillet, crispy-side up, a poached egg and lashings of hollandaise sauce. Sprinkle with chives to finish and enjoy.

3 tablespoons olive oil

4 shallots, finely diced

1 medium red chilli/chile

100 g/⅔ cup dried haricot or
cannellini beans, soaked overnight
with fresh bay leaves and garlic

3 tablespoons white wine

500 ml/2 cups chicken stock

4 x hake fillets (each weighing about
175 g/6 oz.), skin on

75 g/3 oz. padrón peppers

80 g/⅔ cup diced gluten-free chorizo

a generous bunch of fresh flat-leaf
parsley, chopped

grated zest and freshly squeezed juice
of 2 lemons

30 g/2 tablespoons unsalted butter

2 garlic cloves, crushed

sea salt and freshly ground black
pepper

serves 4

The padrón peppers and spicy chorizo complement the hake
magnificently and create a truly tasty comforting Spanish dish,
that is still ideal for any informal supper party.

roasted hake with white beans & padrón peppers

Heat 1 tablespoon of the olive oil in a medium, non-stick frying pan/
skillet. Add the shallots and chilli/chile and cook over a medium heat.
Add the drained soaked beans and white wine and reduce the wine by
half. Then add the chicken stock and cook for 45 minutes until the beans
are tender. Add more liquid if necessary. Season with salt and pepper.

Heat a heavy-based frying pan/skillet and add 1 tablespoon of the olive
oil. Season the hake with salt and pepper and place skin-side down in
the pan. Cook for about 4 minutes, until the skin is crispy. Turn and cook
for a further 3 minutes. Remove from the heat and cover the pan with foil.

Heat the remaining olive oil in a second pan. Add the padrón peppers,
chorizo, parsley, lemon zest and juice, butter and garlic. Cook for about
2 minutes until the peppers are wilted.

When you are ready to serve, spoon the cooked beans onto the middle of
warmed plates. Top with the hake and spoon over the padrón peppers
and chorizo mixture. If you want, you can serve with plenty of crusty
gluten-free bread for mopping up the juices.

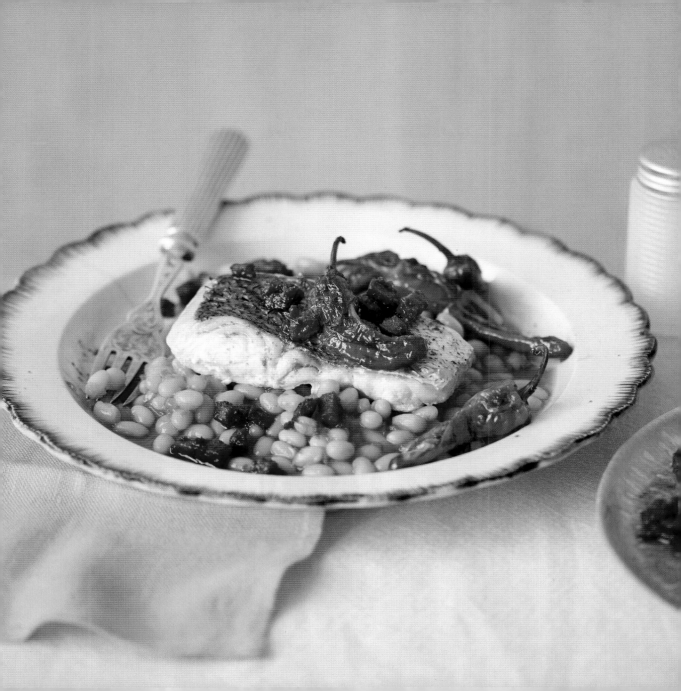

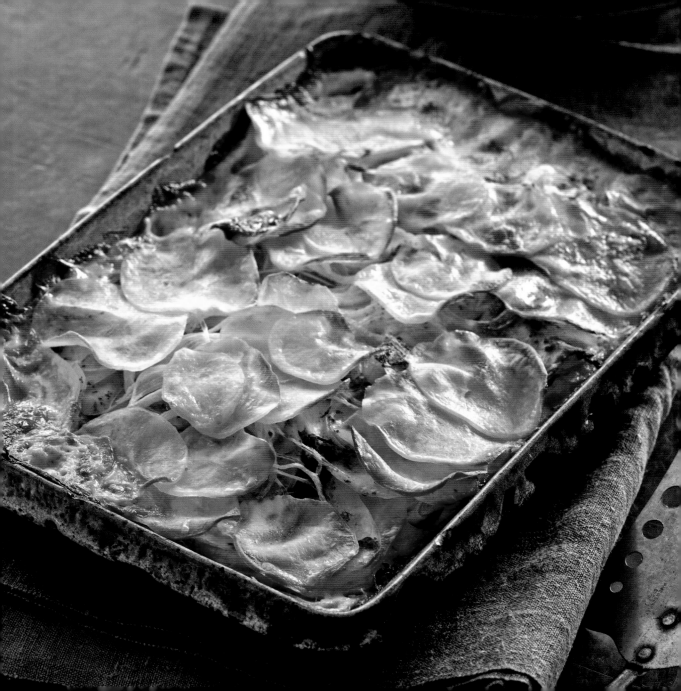

anchovy & potato gratin

The strong saltiness of canned anchovies is used in an unusual way to deliver a satisfying hearty dish that can be served on its own with a salad, or as an accompaniment to roast lamb or pork.

150 g/1½ cups spinach

55 g/2 oz. canned anchovies

4 garlic cloves, peeled

6 roasting potatoes, peeled

3 brown onions, peeled

300 ml/1¼ cups double/heavy cream

a 20 x 25-cm/8 x 10-in. casserole dish

serves 4

Preheat the oven to 160°C (325°F) Gas 3.

Put the spinach and 50 ml/3½ tablespoons of water in a saucepan over a medium heat. Cover and cook until steam forms, then remove from the heat. Transfer the wilted spinach and its cooking liquor to a food processor and add the anchovies and garlic, then blend to a purée. Set aside.

In the food processor using a slicing blade, very thinly slice the potatoes, but do not rinse the potatoes after they have been sliced as the starch binds the dish together. Very thinly slice the onions in the same way. You can hone your knife skills and cut them by hand if you prefer.

Arrange a thin layer of potatoes on the base of the casserole dish. Using a pastry brush or with a spoon, thinly coat the potato layer with the anchovy, garlic and spinach purée. Next, add a very thin layer of onions. Repeat this layering process as many times as possible, finishing with a layer of potatoes. Ensure there is enough room left at the top of the dish for expansion while cooking (about 1 cm/½ in.).

Pour over most of the cream and leave it to settle for 10 minutes, before adding more cream until the top is just covered. Cover with foil and bake in the preheated oven for 1½ hours. Check the cooking after 1 hour, then at 15 minute intervals – a knife should cut through all the layers easily and if the potato is soft, the gratin is ready.

Remove the foil and place back in the oven, increasing the temperature to 180°C (350°F) Gas 4 for 10 minutes, to brown the top. Slice and serve the gratin like you would a lasagne.

Note
You can store the cooked gratin in the fridge for up to 4 days but do not crisp at the higher temperature. To reheat from chilled, bake at 180°C (350°F) Gas 4 for 25 minutes.

100 g/¾ cup cornflour/cornstarch

500 g/1 lb. cod fillets, skin removed
and cut into sixteen 2.5 x 10 cm/
1 x 4 inch fingers

2 eggs, beaten

250 g/2½ cups gluten-free
breadcrumbs

vegetable oil, for frying

for the mayonnaise

2 egg yolks

1 garlic clove, crushed

1 tablespoon freshly squeezed
lemon juice

large pinch of sea salt

300 ml/1¼ cups good-quality extra
virgin olive oil and 300 ml/1¼ cups
sunflower oil, mixed together

for the mushy peas

extra virgin olive oil

½ onion, finely chopped

500 g/1 lb. shelled peas

1–2 garlic cloves, peeled

handful of fresh mint leaves

grated zest of ½ lemon, plus the
whole lemon cut into wedges, to serve

sea salt and freshly ground black
pepper

serves 4

cod fish fingers with mushy peas & mayonnaise

These home-made fish fingers may take a while to make, but they are well worth the effort. The mushy peas can be made with garden peas but purists will choose traditional marrowfat peas.

To make the mayonnaise, you can use a food processor or whisk it by hand. Either way start off with all the ingredients in a bowl, apart from the oil. As you start to process/whisk, very slowly feed in the oil a little at a time until the mixture begins to emulsify and come together. Once this happens you can add the oil in a bit faster, but don't be tempted to pour it in too quickly or it will split. Adding a few drops of boiling water when it looks like it might split usually brings it back together. When all the oil is blended in, taste, and if necessary, adjust the seasoning with a little more lemon juice and salt. Cover and refrigerate until needed.

To make the mushy peas, first place a frying pan/skillet over a medium heat with 1 tablespoon of olive oil, add in the chopped onion and sauté for 10 minutes until translucent, making sure not to let them colour. Keep to one side. Bring a large saucepan of water to the boil. Add in the peas and boil for 4 minutes or until completely tender. Drain the peas and add most of them to a food processor with the onion, garlic, mint, lemon zest and 1 teaspoon of salt. Blitz the mixture, pouring in 1 tablespoon of olive oil at a time until you have a thick purée consistency. Remove to a bowl and stir in the remaining whole peas. Adjust seasoning with salt, pepper and a little more olive oil if necessary.

For the fish fingers, in a bowl combine the cornflour/cornstarch with 1 teaspoon salt and plenty of black pepper. Cover each cod finger in flour, then beaten egg and finally roll in the breadcrumbs until evenly covered. Pour about 1 cm/½ inch of vegetable oil into a frying pan/skillet and place over a medium-high heat. When hot, fry the cod fingers in batches for about 2½ minutes on each side until crisp and golden. Remove, drain and keep warm. To serve, spoon mushy peas onto a plate and arrange the cod fingers on top, with lemon wedges and the mayonnaise for dunking.

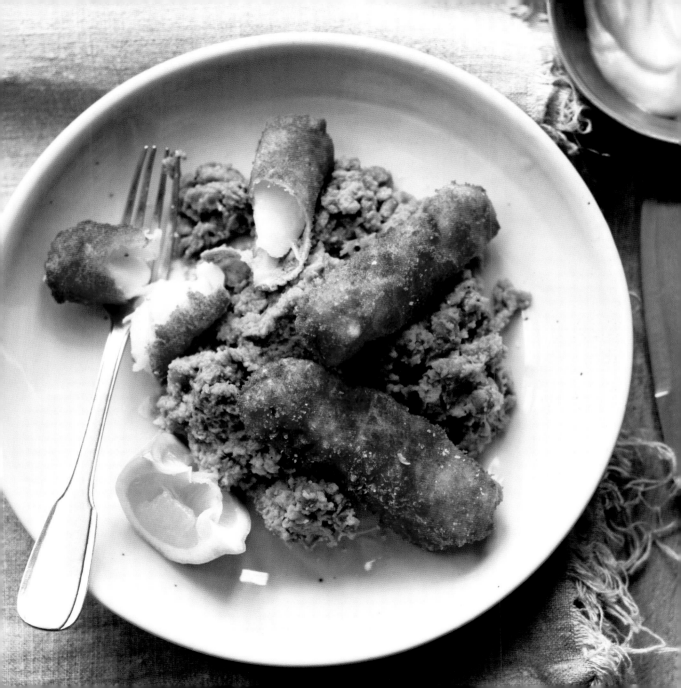

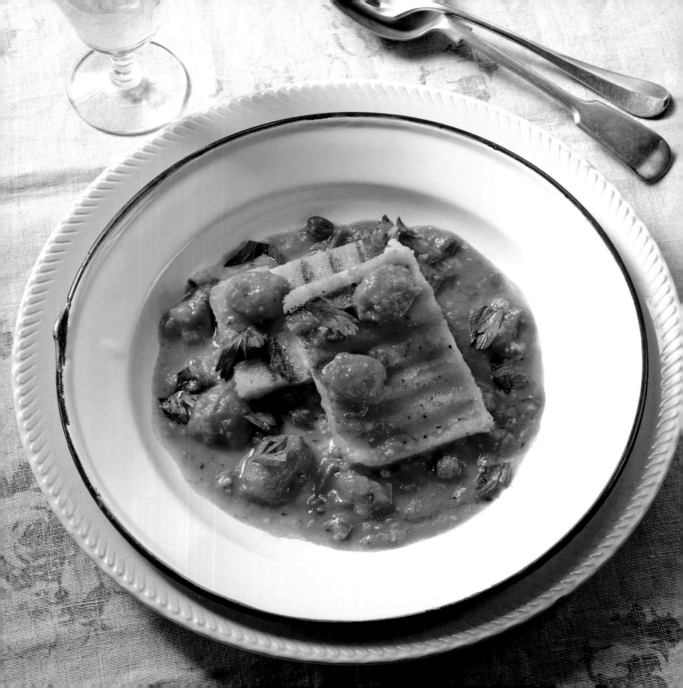

A feisty, spicy Italian tomato sauce contrasts nicely with the comforting blandness of griddled polenta in this hearty dish.

polenta puttanesca

200 g/1⅓ cups instant polenta

sea salt and freshly ground black pepper

for the puttanesca sauce

2 tablespoons olive oil

1 garlic clove, chopped

6 anchovy fillets in oil, drained and chopped

800 g/1¾ lbs. canned peeled cherry tomatoes

2 small dried chillies/chiles, finely chopped

2 teaspoons capers, rinsed

2 generous pinches of dried oregano

chopped fresh flat-leaf parsley, to garnish

a 23-cm/9-in. square baking pan, greased

a ridged stove-top griddle/grill pan

serves 4

First, prepare the polenta. Put the polenta and 800 ml/3⅓ cups of cold water in a large saucepan or pot and season well with salt. Set over a medium-high heat and bring to the boil, stirring continuously. Reduce the heat and simmer, stirring often, until the polenta thickens and begins to come away from the sides of the pan. Transfer to the prepared baking pan, patting smooth with the back of a spoon and set aside to cool.

While the polenta is cooling, prepare the puttanesca sauce. Heat the olive oil in a large frying pan/skillet set over a medium heat. Add the garlic and fry until fragrant. Then add the anchovy fillets and fry until they melt in the pan. Mix in the cherry tomatoes, dried chillies/chiles, capers and oregano and season with pepper. Cook, stirring often, for 15–20 minutes, until the sauce has reduced and thickened.

Preheat the oven to 110°C (225°F) Gas ¼.

Cut the cooled, set polenta into eight even-sized squares.

Preheat the griddle/grill pan until very hot, then cook the polenta in batches until marked by the griddle on each side, keeping each square warm in the preheated oven.

Gently heat through the puttanesca sauce over a low heat, then spoon over the griddled polenta squares and sprinkle over the parsley, to serve.

Chicken cacciatore translates as 'hunter's chicken'. Classic Italian ingredients, including tomatoes, garlic and wine, are transformed into a thick, tasty sauce that coats the fried chicken. Serve with mashed potatoes, rice or polenta.

chicken cacciatore

600 g/1 lb. 5 oz. ripe tomatoes

4 chicken drumsticks

4 chicken thighs

plain/all-purpose gluten-free flour, to coat

3 tablespoons olive oil

1 rasher/strip of pancetta, diced

2 garlic cloves, chopped

4 fresh rosemary sprigs

1 yellow (bell) pepper, deseeded and sliced into strips

75 ml/scant ⅓ cup dry white wine

1 tablespoon tomato purée/paste

sea salt and freshly ground black pepper

serves 4

Begin by scalding the tomatoes. Pour boiling water over the tomatoes in a heatproof bowl. Set aside for 1 minute, then drain and carefully peel off the skins using a sharp knife. Roughly chop, reserving any juices, and set aside.

Season the chicken pieces with salt and pepper, then season the flour with salt and pepper in a wide, shallow dish. Coat the chicken pieces in the seasoned flour, ready to fry.

In a large frying pan/skillet, heat 2 tablespoons of the oil. Fry the chicken in batches, until golden-brown on all sides.

Heat the remaining oil in a casserole dish. Add the pancetta and garlic and fry, stirring occasionally, for 1–2 minutes, until the garlic is lightly browned. Add the rosemary and the (bell) pepper and fry for 1 minute. Pour in the wine and cook, stirring occasionally, for 1–2 minutes, until the wine has reduced slightly. Add the chopped tomatoes with their juices, cover and cook for 5 minutes, until the sauce has come to the boil. Stir well, to help the tomatoes break down, then stir in the tomato purée/paste. Season with salt and pepper and simmer uncovered for 10 minutes, stirring from time to time.

Add the browned chicken pieces to the tomato sauce. Bring to the boil, reduce the heat and simmer, partly covered, for 20–30 minutes, until the chicken is cooked through. Serve.

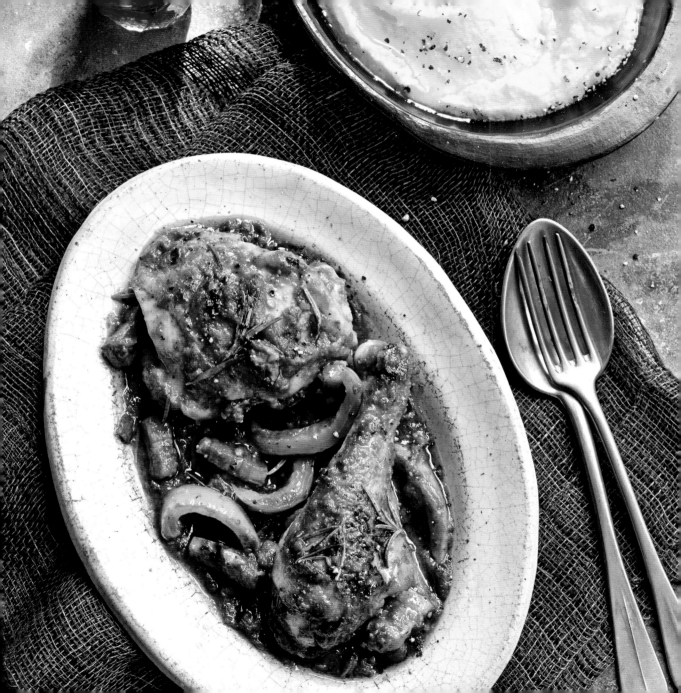

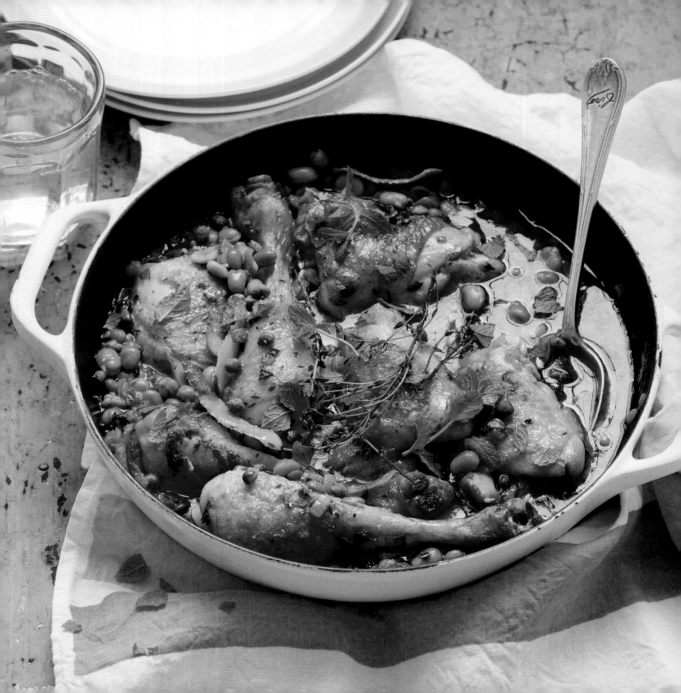

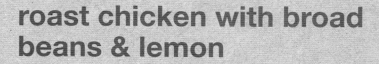

roast chicken with broad beans & lemon

375 g/2½ cups fresh shelled broad/fava beans

2 tablespoons olive oil

1.5 kg/3 lb. 5 oz. chicken portions, bone in, skin on

3 onions, roughly chopped

a handful of fresh thyme

grated zest and freshly squeezed juice of 2 lemons

3 garlic cloves, thinly sliced

350 ml/1½ cups fresh chicken stock

a handful of fresh mint leaves

2 tablespoons capers, rinsed

sea salt and freshly ground black pepper

serves 4

This chicken dish is tasty, colourful and earthy and makes a perfect relaxed, easy summer Sunday roast. It tastes simply divine when served with a lemon and parsley mash.

Preheat the oven to 200°C (400°F) Gas 6.

Bring a pan of water to the boil. Add the broad/fava beans and boil for 2 minutes. Drain and refresh under cold running water. Peel away the skins and discard.

Heat the oil in a casserole dish over a high heat. Cook the chicken portions in two batches, for 4 minutes on each side until browned. Remove from the dish and set aside.

Add the onions, thyme and lemon zest to the casserole dish and cook for 2 minutes. Return the chicken and any juices to the dish with the garlic and stock. Bring to the boil, and add salt and pepper. Transfer to the oven and cook, uncovered, for 40 minutes.

Stir in the broad/fava beans and 2 tablespoons of lemon juice and top with mint and capers. Season with salt and pepper to taste and serve.

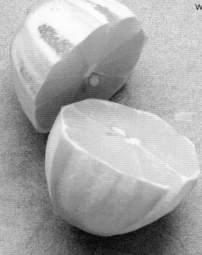

4 chicken thighs and 4 wings

extra virgin olive oil

sea salt

1 tablespoon ras el hanout (spice mix)

1 teaspoon dried chilli/hot red pepper flakes

1 red onion, halved and thinly sliced

1 teaspoon ground cinnamon

1 teaspoon ground cumin

3 garlic cloves, crushed

250 g/1¼ cups quinoa

12 dried apricots, sliced

grated zest of ½ lemon

a handful each of fresh flat-leaf parsley, mint and coriander/cilantro leaves, chopped, plus extra to serve

1 tablespoon pomegranate molasses, or lemon juice

freshly ground black pepper

rose petals (optional)

serves 4–6

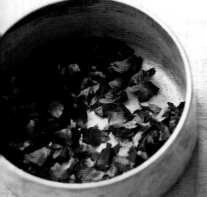

spiced chicken with quinoa, lemon zest & rose petals

Quinoa is a great base for salads or served as it is here, spiced up and served with meat or fish. It's a fantastic source of protein, containing all the essential amino acids, and can be used in the same way as couscous. The rose petals are a lovely addition and do certainly add flavour, but it is subtle, so feel free to omit if you like. For a vegetarian version, swap the chicken for roasted squash, and use vegetable stock instead.

Preheat the oven to 190°C (375°F) Gas 5.

Place the chicken in a large roasting pan and drizzle over 1 tablespoon of olive oil, just enough to coat them. Season with plenty of salt and sprinkle over the ras el hanout and chilli/hot red pepper flakes. Use your hands to massage the spices into the chicken. Roast for 25–30 minutes or until cooked through and the skin is crisp and golden. Keep warm.

In a large saucepan, gently sauté the red onion in a little olive oil until soft. Add in the cinnamon, cumin, garlic and 1 teaspoon salt and fry for another couple of minutes until aromatic. Add in the quinoa and just under double its quantity of water, about 500 ml/2 cups. Bring to the boil, then reduce the heat to low and place the lid on top. Cook for about 12 minutes, then remove the lid and continue to cook until all the water has been absorbed and the quinoa is quite dry. Turn off the heat and add in the sliced apricots and lemon zest. Stir in the herbs, pomegranate molasses (or lemon juice), and season to taste with salt and pepper. Gently combine together.

Plate up the quinoa with the chicken on top and remaining herbs and rose petals scattered over.

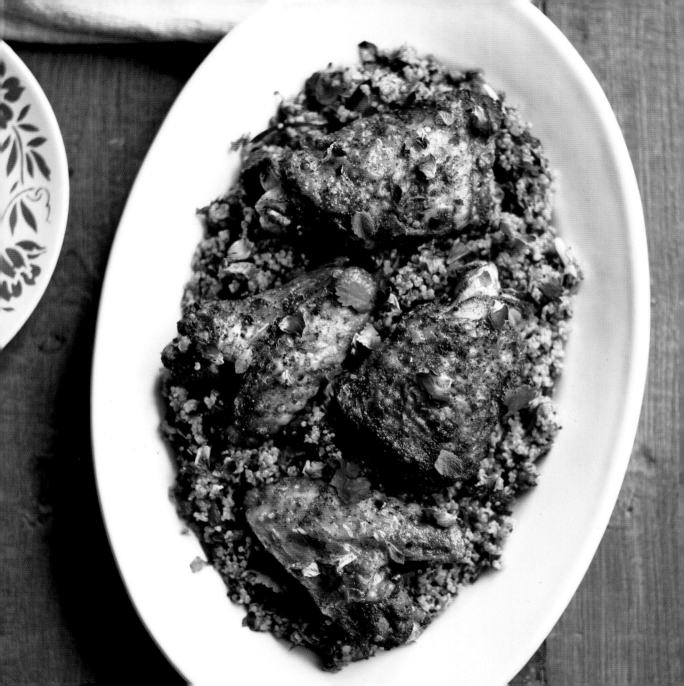

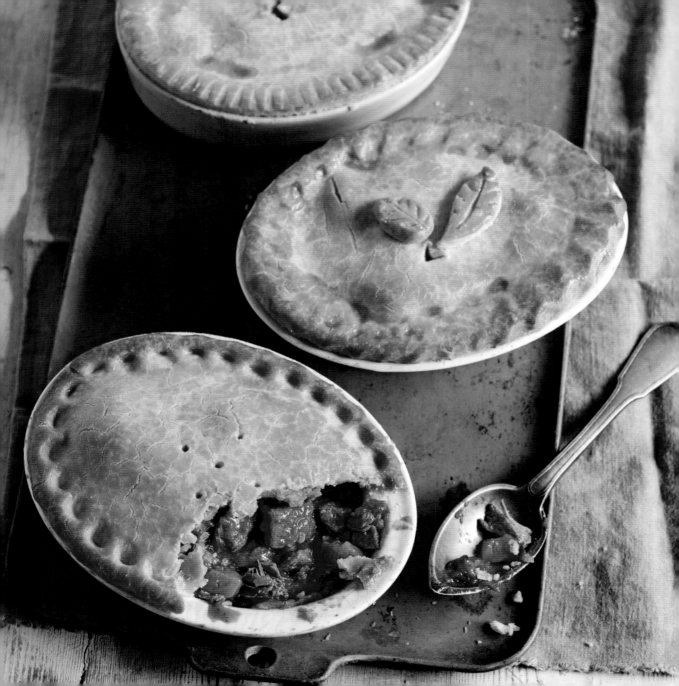

Those who avoid gluten usually have to avoid 'ale' and 'pie' when eating out, but at home it's different. This tasty recipe uses both.

steak & ale pies

800 g/1¾ lb. casserole/chuck steak, in chunks

3 tablespoons plain/all-purpose gluten-free flour

2 teaspoons sea salt

2 teaspoons ground white pepper

2–3 tablespoons vegetable or olive oil

1 onion, chopped

2 garlic cloves, finely chopped

4 carrots, chopped

4 large celery sticks, chopped

a 330-ml/12-oz. bottle of gluten-free ale

1 tablespoon tomato purée/paste

1 tablespoon balsamic vinegar

400 ml/1⅔ cups gluten-free beef stock

1 batch Hot Water Pastry (see page 67), refrigerated

1 egg, beaten

4 x 500-ml/18-oz. pie dishes

makes 4 individual pies

To make the filling, toss the steak pieces with the flour, salt and pepper. Heat 2 tablespoons of oil in a large lidded casserole dish or frying pan/skillet and fry the meat for a few minutes until browned on all sides. Remove with a slotted spoon and set aside. Add the onion and garlic with a little more oil to the pan and sauté until the onion is soft. Stir in the remaining vegetables and cook for a few minutes longer, then lift out of the pan and set aside with the meat. Deglaze the pan with a large glug of ale, scraping up any crusty bits from the bottom and stirring into the liquid. Add the remaining ale and bring to a simmer. Stir in the tomato purée and balsamic vinegar, then return the meat and vegetables to the pan. Pour over the stock and give everything a stir. Bring to the boil, turn down the heat, cover and simmer for 2 hours. Remove the lid, stir and simmer for a further 30 minutes, uncovered, before removing from the heat and setting aside to cool for 1–2 hours. When the filling has cooled down and you're ready to bake the pies, preheat the oven to 200°C (400°F) Gas 6.

Take the pastry from the fridge. Divide into eight pieces and roll each piece into a ball with your hands. Put all but one piece back into the fridge. Lay a piece of clingfilm/plastic wrap onto the work surface. Put the pastry piece in the middle and lay a second piece of clingfilm/plastic wrap over the top. Roll out the pastry to an oval or circle larger than the pie dishes, to a thickness of 2–3 mm/⅛ inch. Remove the top layer of clingfilm/plastic wrap and, using the layer underneath to help you, lift and turn over the pastry into the pie dish to line it. Press gently into the corners – try not to break it. Remove the clingfilm/plastic wrap, set aside and repeat.

Fill each lined dish with the cooled filling. Take the remaining pastry from the fridge and roll out to create four lids. Press each lid onto the overhanging pastry lining the dishes and then trim the excess with a sharp knife and make decorative leaves if you wish. Cut a small vent in the top of each pie dish and then brush the tops with the beaten egg. Bake in the preheated oven for 25–30 minutes until golden and the filling is piping hot.

500 g/1 lb. 2 oz. tomatoes

2 tablespoons olive oil

1 onion, chopped

2 garlic cloves, chopped

a 5-cm/2-in. piece of fresh ginger, peeled and finely chopped

2 cardamom pods

1 cinnamon stick

1 bay leaf

500 g/1 lb. 2 oz. minced/ground lamb or beef

1 teaspoon sea salt

⅓ teaspoon ground turmeric

2 teaspoons ground cumin

2 teaspoons ground coriander

1 teaspoon freshly ground black pepper

steamed rice, to serve

serves 4

Fragrant spices enhance the flavour of the tomatoes to make an aromatic sauce for these punchy spiced meatballs. For a wholesome meal, serve them with steamed rice and natural/plain yogurt on the side.

meatballs in spiced tomato sauce

Begin by scalding the tomatoes. Pour boiling water over the tomatoes in a heatproof bowl. Set aside for 1 minute, then drain and carefully peel off the skins using a sharp knife. Roughly chop, reserving any juices and set aside.

Heat 1 tablespoon of the oil in a large, heavy-bottomed saucepan or casserole dish set over a medium heat. Add the onion, half the garlic, the ginger, cardamom pods, cinnamon stick and bay leaf. Fry for 1–2 minutes, stirring often, until fragrant. Add the chopped tomatoes with their juices, cover and bring to the boil. Once boiling, uncover and cook for 10 minutes, stirring now and then to break down the tomatoes so that they form a sauce.

Make the meatballs by mixing together the meat, the remaining garlic, the salt, ground turmeric, cumin and coriander, and pepper in a large mixing bowl. With wet hands, shape the spiced meat into small meatballs, the size of large marbles.

Heat the remaining oil in a large frying pan/skillet. Add the meatballs and fry, stirring occasionally, until browned on all sides.

Transfer the meatballs to the pan or dish with the tomato sauce and bring to the boil. Reduce the heat, half cover and simmer for 20–25 minutes until the meatballs are cooked through and the sauce has reduced. Serve with steamed rice.

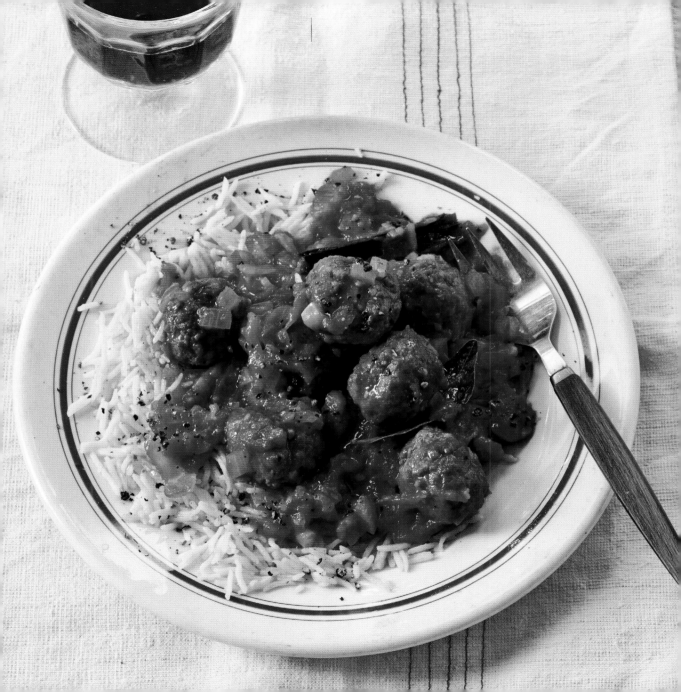

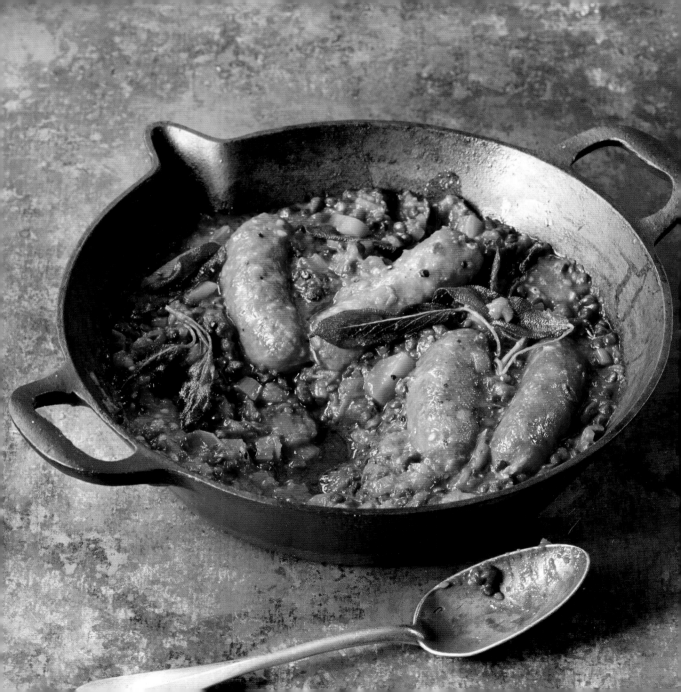

Puy lentils in sage and tomato sauce

200 g/1 cup dried Puy/French green lentils

1 tablespoon olive oil

½ onion, chopped

½ carrot, peeled and sliced

1 celery stick, finely chopped

4 fresh sage leaves, shredded, plus whole leaves to garnish

a glug of red wine

400 g/14 oz. canned peeled plum tomatoes

sea salt and freshly ground black pepper

hot cooked gluten-free pork or vegetarian sausages, to serve (optional)

serves 4 as a side dish, 2 as a main

Tomatoes and lentils are a classic combination. Serve this hearty dish as a side with robust-flavoured meat dishes such as roast pork belly with garlic or beef stews. Or you can serve it as seen here: with gluten-free sausages as a main.

Rinse the lentils under cold, running water. Put them in a saucepan, cover with cold water and bring to the boil over a medium heat. Reduce the heat and simmer for 10–15 minutes, until tender; drain.

Meanwhile, heat the oil in a heavy-bottomed saucepan set over a medium heat. Add the onion, carrot and celery and cook for 2–3 minutes, until softened. Sprinkle over the shredded sage and pour in the wine. Cook briskly for 1 minute before adding the canned tomatoes. Season with salt and pepper and bring to the boil. Reduce the heat and simmer for 15 minutes, stirring now and then to break up the tomatoes.

Mix the drained lentils into the tomato sauce and warm through along with the whole sage leaves. Add the cooked sausages if desired and serve at once.

boeuf bourguignon

This classic French dish is a rich combination of slow-cooked, tender, wine-marinated beef, flavoured with herbs, bacon, mushrooms and garlic. Serve it with creamy mashed potatoes and green beans. As it can be made in advance, this is an ideal comfort dish for entertaining.

800 g/1¾ lb. braising steak, cubed

750 ml/3 cups red wine, ideally Burgundy

1 onion, roughly chopped

1 carrot, roughly chopped

3 garlic cloves, chopped

4 fresh thyme sprigs

2 fresh bay leaves

2 tablespoons olive oil

1 shallot, chopped

2 rashers/slices smoked bacon, chopped into thin strips

400 ml/1¾ cups beef stock

15 g/1 tablespoon butter

200 g/7 oz. button mushrooms

sea salt and freshly ground black pepper

chopped parsley, and creamy mashed potatoes and green beans (optional), to serve

serves 6–8

Place the steak in a large bowl with the red wine, onion, carrot, garlic, thyme and bay leaves and stir, then marinate in the fridge for at least 3 hours, or ideally overnight.

Preheat the oven to 150°C (300°F) Gas 2.

Remove the beef from the marinade and pat dry with paper towels. Discard the onion and carrot, but reserve the rest of the red wine marinade (i.e. the garlic and herbs). Place the reserved marinade in a pan, bring to the boil and cook uncovered until reduced to about 600 ml/2½ cups.

Heat 1 tablespoon of the olive oil in the casserole dish. Add the beef and fry for 3–5 minutes until browned on all sides. Set aside.

Wipe out the casserole dish with paper towels. Add the remaining olive oil, heat through and fry the shallot and bacon for 1–2 minutes, until fragrant. Add the browned beef, reduced red wine and the beef stock. Season with salt and pepper. Bring to the boil, cover and cook in the preheated oven for 2 hours.

Towards the end of the casserole's cooking time, heat the butter in a frying pan/skillet and fry the mushrooms until golden brown. Stir the mushrooms into the casserole and serve garnished with chopped parsley, and creamy mashed potatoes and green beans, if liked.

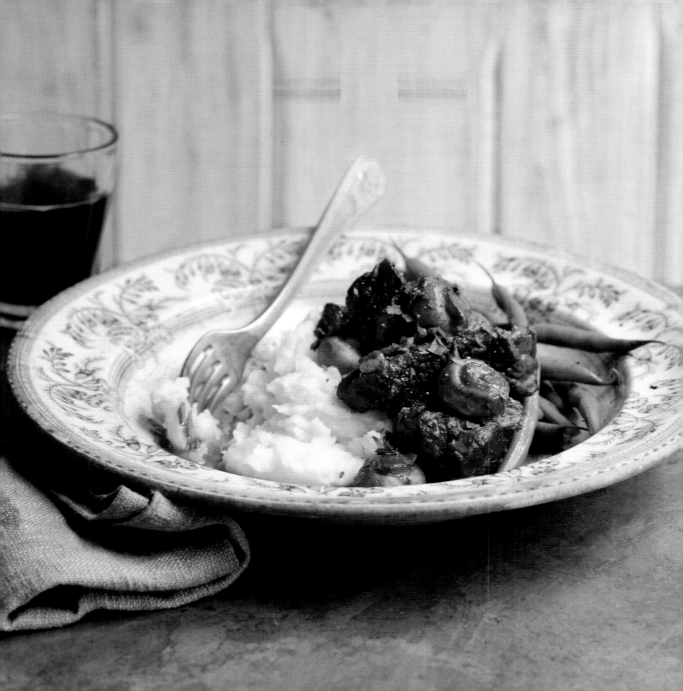

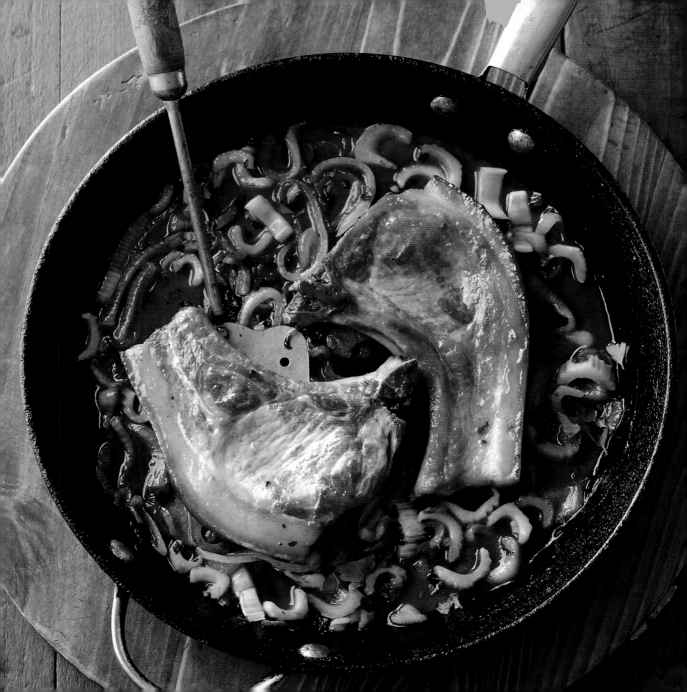

pork stroganoff

15 g/1 tablespoon butter

1 small white onion, diced

1 garlic clove, chopped

110 g/1 ½ cups mushrooms, sliced

200 g/7 oz. pork shoulder, diced

1 teaspoon wholegrain mustard

a pinch of freshly chopped parsley

a pinch of freshly chopped tarragon

4 tablespoons double/heavy cream

1 tablespoon brandy

mashed potatoes and some green vegetables, to serve

sea salt and freshly ground black pepper

serves 2

Such an easy one-pot dish and a great use of pork shoulder. It's great with all the easiest accompaniments like rice, potatoes or gluten-free pasta, so it's a perfect one to make in a larger batch and freeze in portions for easy lunches and dinners.

Melt the butter in a pan over a medium heat and fry the onion, garlic and mushrooms until they start to brown. Add a pinch of salt and pepper, then the diced pork. Continue to fry for 4–5 minutes to cook the pork through.

Stir in the mustard, parsley, tarragon, cream and brandy. Reduce the heat to low, pop a lid on top and simmer. For this two-portion quantity, it will only need 15–20 minutes; for a larger batch, double the time and just give it a stir occasionally until the sauce thickens.

Serve hot with mashed potatoes and greens seasoned to taste with salt and pepper.

Note
You can cool the mixture right down and portion in sealed containers or sandwich bags and freeze for up to 3 months.

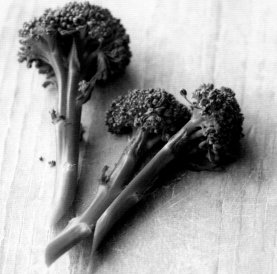

shepherd's pie

600 g/1 lb. 5 oz. all-purpose potatoes, such as Maris Piper or Yukon Gold, peeled and chopped into 2.5-cm/1-inch chunks

45 g/3 tablespoons butter

1 garlic clove, crushed

2 carrots, chopped

1 white onion, chopped

500 g/1 lb. 2 oz. lamb mince/ground lamb

20 g/4 teaspoons tomato purée/paste

200 ml/scant 1 cup red wine

150 ml/⅔ cup vegetable stock

a pinch of dried rosemary

a pinch of dried thyme

40 g/generous ⅓ cup rolled oats

50 ml/3½ tablespoons milk

20 g/⅓ cup finely grated Parmesan cheese, plus extra for sprinkling on top (optional)

sea salt and freshly ground black pepper

a 20 x 25-cm/8 x 10-inch ovenproof dish, greased

serves 4

Shepherd's pie uses minced/ground lamb, whereas cottage pie uses minced/ground beef – and this comforting pie is lovely with either. The oats help to make the mixture soft and squishy but stop it from going slimy, which flour can sometimes do when you use it to thicken the base of a pie.

Preheat the oven to 180°C (350°F) Gas 4.

Bring a large pan of water to the boil and boil the potatoes for about 20 minutes, until soft enough to mash.

Meanwhile, heat 15 g/1 tablespoon of the butter in a frying pan/skillet over a medium heat and add the garlic, carrots and onion. Fry for about 4–5 minutes, until softened and starting to brown.

Add the lamb and fry until browned all over, breaking it up as it cooks using a wooden spoon.

Add the tomato purée/paste and stir in. Then add the red wine, vegetable stock, rosemary, thyme and some salt and pepper. Stir well and then add the oats, a little at a time. Mix well and cook, stirring, until the mixture is nice and thick and the oats have absorbed the liquid.

By now the potatoes should be soft, so drain and mash them, mixing in the milk, Parmesan and remaining 30 g/2 tablespoons of butter.

Spoon the lamb mixture into the greased ovenproof dish and press down to make it level. Then spread the mashed potatoes evenly over the top.

Put the dish in the preheated oven and bake for 20 minutes. To brown the top, add a little more Parmesan (or sprinkle with grated mature Cheddar) and place under a hot grill/broiler for the last 5 minutes.

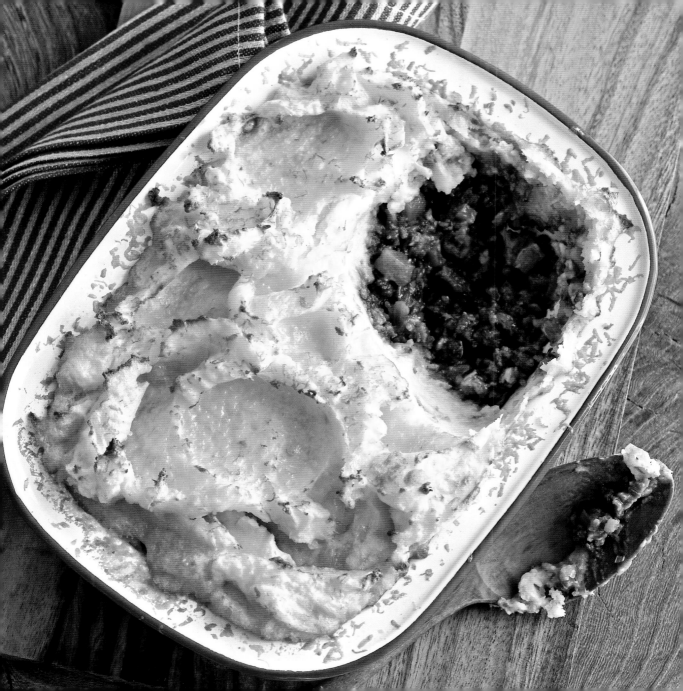

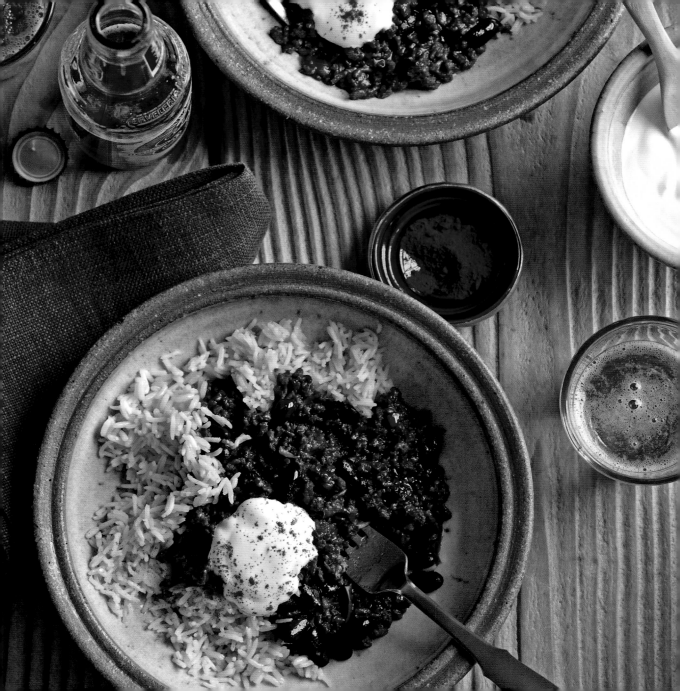

2 tablespoons olive oil

1 red onion, finely chopped

1 garlic clove, finely chopped

800 g/1 lb. 12 oz. minced/ground beef

1 chilli/chile, deseeded and finely chopped

a pinch of cayenne pepper, plus extra to serve

a pinch of ground cumin

a pinch of ground coriander

2 teaspoons dark muscovado/molasses sugar

1 tablespoon plain/all-purpose gluten-free flour

a pinch each of sea salt and freshly ground black pepper

½ beef stock/bouillon cube (or 30 g/1 oz. veal stock)

1 x 400-g/14-oz. can kidney beans, drained and rinsed (drained weight 250 g/9 oz.)

1 tablespoon tomato purée/paste

100 ml/⅓ cup red wine

200 g/7 oz. canned chopped tomatoes

cooked rice and soured cream, to serve

serves 4

A great and comforting recipe to make in a large batch and freeze in portions. After a quick bit of prep, you can leave this bubbling on the hob/stovetop for as long as you like. It's a good one for the budget, too, with minced/ground beef, kidney beans and chopped tomatoes, all being inexpensive ingredients to buy.

chilli con carne

Heat the oil in a saucepan or deep frying pan/skillet over a medium heat and fry the onion and garlic for about 4–5 minutes until they start to brown. Add the minced/ground beef and fry for another minute, using a wooden spoon to break up the meat.

Add the chilli/chile, cayenne pepper, cumin, coriander, sugar, flour and salt and pepper, and stir until it forms a paste. Then slowly crumble in the beef stock/bouillon cube or add the veal stock. Add the kidney beans, tomato purée/paste, red wine and chopped tomatoes and bring to the boil. Once it bubbles, reduce the heat to low and let it simmer for 45 minutes, or up to an hour if you can, so that it thickens.

Serve straight away with hot rice, a dollop of soured cream and a pinch of cayenne pepper on the top.

Note
Chilli/chili con carne freezes brilliantly: portion it into freezerproof containers or sandwich bags and freeze for up to 3 months. Once defrosted and reheated until piping hot, just check the flavours and add a little chilli/chili powder, salt or cayenne pepper to liven it up a bit, if necessary.

Simple and easy, this steak supper is a great way to get a protein fix at the end of a long day. Buy the best quality meat you can afford – the better the steak, the more delicious the meal.

lemon thyme & pink peppercorn steak

1 sweet potato, cut into wedges

1 sirloin steak

leaves from 6–10 sprigs of fresh lemon thyme, chopped

½–1 tablespoon pink peppercorns, crushed

olive oil, to drizzle

sea salt and freshly ground black pepper

mixed green salad and garlic mayonnaise, to serve

a baking sheet lined with baking parchment

a ridged stove-top griddle/grill pan

serves 1

Preheat the oven to 180°C (350°F) Gas 4.

First prepare the sweet potato wedges. Spread the wedges out on the prepared baking sheet and sprinkle with a little salt. Bake in the preheated oven for 25–30 minutes, or until crisp on the outside and cooked through.

Rub the steak with generous amounts of lemon thyme and crushed pink peppercorns. Season and drizzle with a little oil. Allow the meat to come to room temperature while marinating in this mixture.

Set the griddle/grill pan over medium-high heat until smoking hot. Sear the fat of the steak first, then cook both sides. How well you like it cooked will determine the cooking time (this is also dependent on how thick the steak is): for medium-rare, cook it for 2 minutes on each side.

Remove the steak from the pan, pour over any juices that were released into the pan, and rest for a few minutes before serving with the sweet potato wedges. Serve with a simple mixed salad on the side with a little garlic mayonnaise to dip the sweet potato wedges into.

Note
You can make an easy garlic mayonnaise by stirring crushed garlic through plain mayonnaise (see the Mayonnaise recipe on page 110).

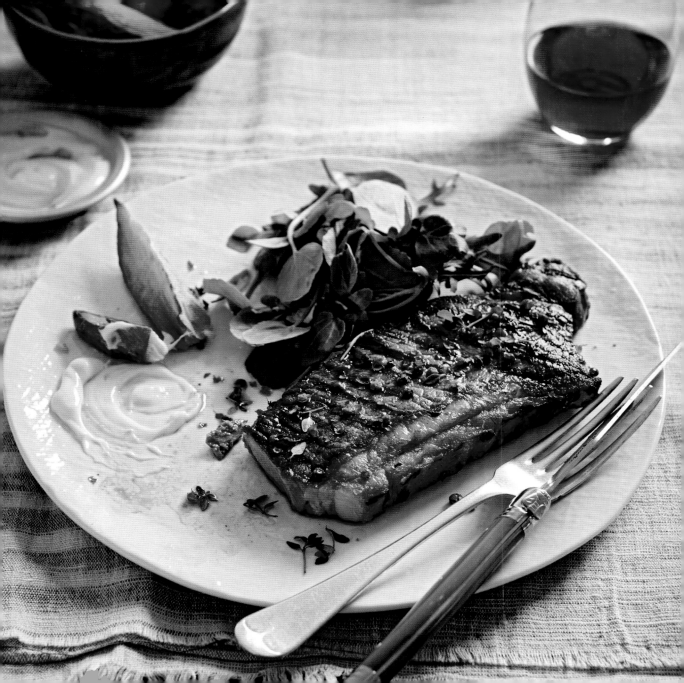

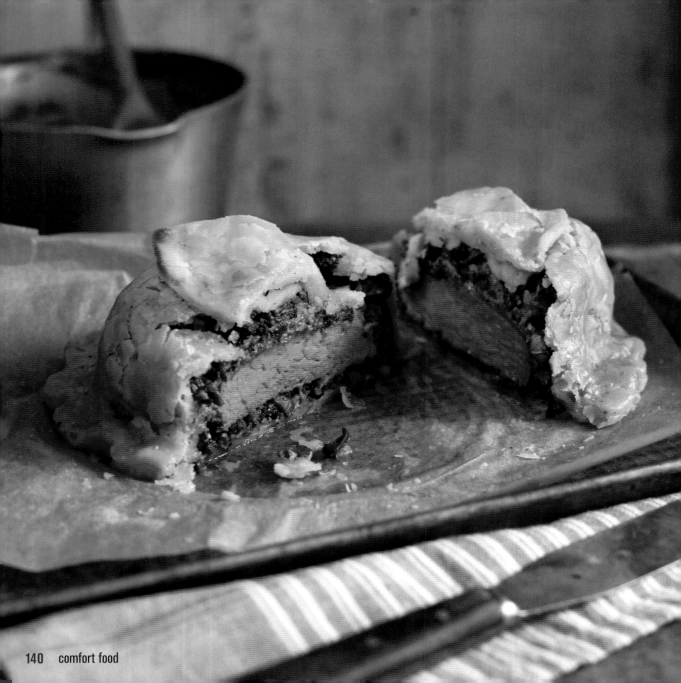

for the mushroom duxelles

25 g/1 oz. dried wild mushrooms

60 ml/¼ cup sweet sherry

50 g/3½ tablespoons butter

55 g/2 oz. girolles mushrooms, finely chopped

55 g/2 oz. trompettes de la mort mushrooms, finely chopped

85 g/3 oz. chestnut mushrooms, finely chopped

truffle salt (or sea salt and a little truffle oil)

freshly ground black pepper

for the pastry

200 g/1⅔ cups plain/all-purpose gluten-free flour, plus extra for dusting

100 g/3½ oz. gluten-free shredded suet OR 6½ tablespoons vegetable shortening, chilled and grated

sea salt and freshly ground black pepper

to assemble

freshly ground black pepper

2 fillet steaks (about 125 g/4½ oz. each)

brandy, for brushing

100 g/3½ oz. gluten-free pork and mushroom pâté

1 egg

2 teaspoons gluten-free Dijon mustard

a ridged stove-top griddle/grill pan

a baking sheet, greased and lined with baking parchment

serves 2

beef Wellingtons

Filled with fillet steak, pâté, mushroom duxelles and a little brandy, these Wellingtons are great for special occasions.

For the duxelles, cover the dried mushrooms in boiling water, add the sherry and leave to soak for about 20 minutes. Once rehydrated, drain the mushrooms, squeeze out any liquid, then finely chop them. Melt the butter in a large frying pan/skillet and add the chopped fresh and rehydrated mushrooms. Season with truffle salt and pepper. Cook the mushrooms until very soft and reduced, then leave to cool completely.

Sprinkle cracked black pepper over the steaks and sear in the hot griddle/grill pan for about 30 seconds on each side. Using kitchen tongs, brown the sides of the steaks, too, so that the meat is sealed all over. Transfer to a plate to cool. Brush with a tablespoon of brandy and chill until needed.

For the pastry, put the flour and suet/vegetable shortening in a large mixing bowl, season with salt and pepper, then gradually add enough water (about 120–150 ml/½–⅔ cup) to bring the mixture together into a soft dough. On a flour-dusted surface, roll out the dough thinly and cut out 2 circles about 17 cm/7 inches in diameter and 2 about 20 cm/8 inches in diameter. Re-roll the trimmings and cut out leaves to decorate the pies.

Lay the 2 smaller pastry circles on the baking sheet. Place a spoonful of the mushroom mixture in the centre of each and place the steaks on top. Cut the pâté into 2 and place a piece on top of each steak, smoothing down with a knife. Cover the pâté with the rest of the mushrooms, pressing down firmly. Brush around the edges of the small pastry circles with a little cold water. Carefully lift the larger pastry circles to top the steaks and mushrooms, smoothing them down so the pastry sits snugly over the filling. Seal and crimp the edges with your fingers, then trim any excess pastry.

Beat the egg with the mustard and use it to glaze the top of the pies. Arrange the pastry leaves on top and brush them with the egg mixture as well. Chill the Wellingtons in the refrigerator until you are ready to cook. Preheat the oven to 180°C (350°F) Gas 4 and bake the beef Wellingtons for 20–25 minutes until the pastry is golden brown. Serve immediately.

cheese & bacon bread pudding

50 g/3½ tablespoons butter

300 ml/1¼ cups milk

300 ml/1¼ cups double/heavy cream

180 g bacon lardons/1 cup thick-sliced back bacon, cut into cubes

1 onion, finely chopped

140 g (drained weight)/⅔ cup sweetcorn/corn kernels

5 slices gluten-free bread (brown or white)

4 eggs, beaten

85 g/¾ cup grated Cheddar cheese

sea salt and freshly ground black pepper

a 25-cm/10-inch ovenproof dish, greased

serves 4

This is a really satisfying dish that is a meal all on its own. It needs no accompaniment, although you could serve it with a salad, if you wish. Rich and creamy, this is the ultimate comfort food on a cold winter's evening.

Preheat the oven to 180°C (350°F) Gas 4.

Put the butter, milk and cream in a saucepan set over a gentle heat, and heat until the butter has melted. Set aside to cool.

Put the bacon lardons/cubes in a frying pan/skillet and cook for a few minutes until they have released some oil and are lightly golden-brown, then add the onion to the pan and cook until softened. Stir in the sweetcorn/corn kernels and cook for a further 2–3 minutes.

Cut the bread slices into quarters and arrange a layer over the base of the ovenproof dish. Spoon over a little of the bacon and corn mixture, spread evenly, then add another layer of bread. Continue layering the bread and filling mixture until all the ingredients are used.

Season the cooled milk mixture with salt and pepper, then whisk in the eggs. Pour the mixture over the bread filling and sprinkle the cheese over the top. Bake in the preheated oven for 25–30 minutes until golden-brown, then serve.

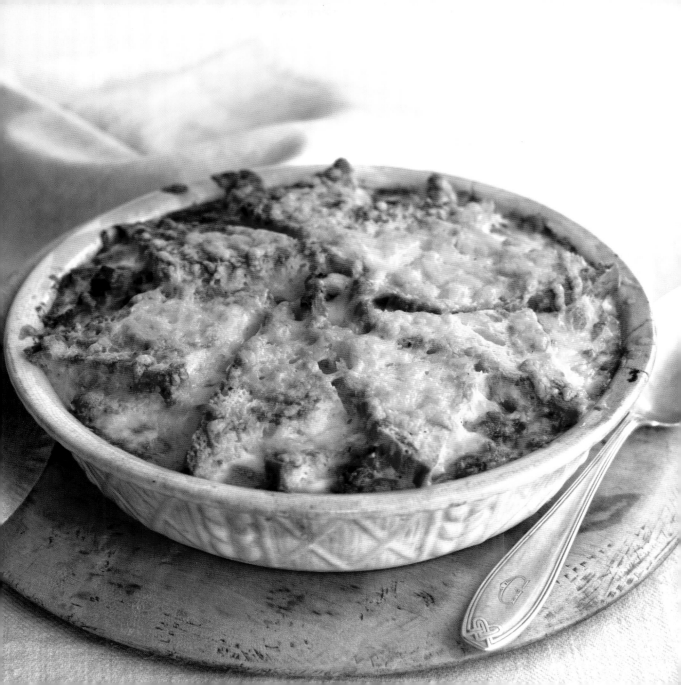

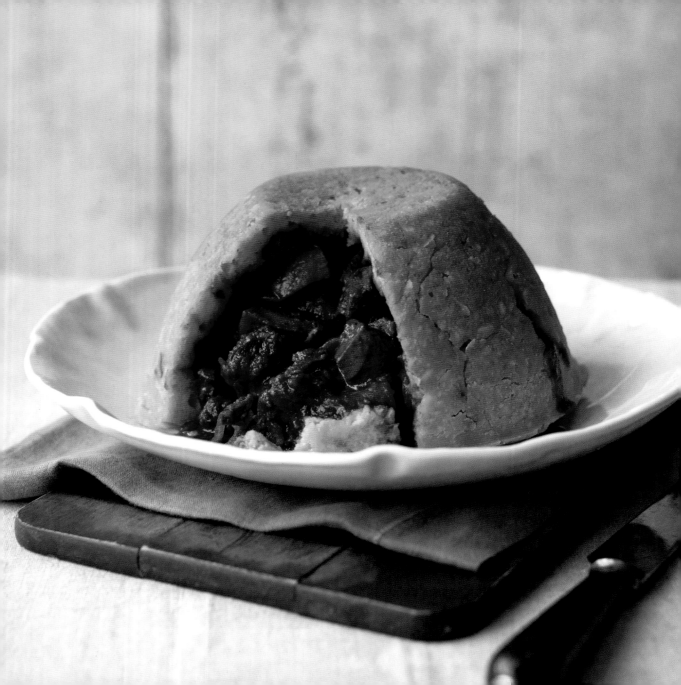

for the filling

1 onion, thinly sliced

1–2 tablespoons olive oil

450 g/1 lb. stewing beef, diced

55 g/2 oz. ox kidneys, chopped

150 ml/⅔ cup medium sweet sherry

120 ml/½ cup beef stock

100 g/3½ oz. baby carrots, trimmed

3 open cap mushrooms, quartered

1 tablespoon cornflour/cornstarch

sea salt and freshly ground black pepper

for the suet crust

225 g/2 cups self-raising/rising gluten-free flour plus 1 teaspoon gluten-free baking powder OR 1¾ cups plain/all-purpose gluten-free flour plus 3 teaspoons gluten-free baking powder and 1½ teaspoons xanthan gum, plus extra flour for dusting

100 g/3½ oz. gluten-free shredded suet OR 6½ tablespoons vegetable shortening, chilled and grated

2 teaspoons gluten-free Dijon mustard

½ teaspoon sea salt

about 250 ml/1 cup milk

a large flameproof lidded casserole

a 900-ml/3½-cup pudding basin, greased

kitchen string

serves 4

Steamed suet pudding is real comfort food. Gluten-free suet pastry works well: suet stops the pastry being crumbly and dry.

steak & kidney pudding

Preheat the oven to 180°C (350°F) Gas 4. To make the filling, cook the onion with the olive oil in the casserole over a gentle heat until it starts to colour. Remove from the pan and set aside. Add the beef to the pan with a little more oil and lightly brown to seal. Add the kidneys and cook, stirring, for 2–3 minutes. Add the sherry and cook for a few minutes, then add the cooked onion, stock, carrots and mushrooms, and season to taste. Transfer the casserole, covered, to the preheated oven and cook for 1 hour, turning the temperature down to 170°C (325°F) Gas 3 after 30 minutes. Remove a few spoonfuls of the juices from the pan, mix well with the cornflour/cornstarch, stir back into the meat to thicken the sauce, then leave to cool.

For the suet crust, put the flour, baking powder (plus xanthan gum, if using), suet/vegetable shortening, mustard and salt in a large mixing bowl and gradually add the milk (you may not need it all) to make a smooth non-sticky dough. On a flour-dusted surface, roll out the pastry to a circle about 25 cm/10 inches in diameter and about 8 mm/⅜ inch thick. Cut away a quarter wedge of the dough circle and set aside. Wet the cut edges with a little water and use the dough to line the pudding basin, pressing the two cut edges together. On a flour-dusted surface, roll the remaining dough into a circle the size of the top of the pudding basin. Spoon the cooled meat mixture into the basin. Wet the top edge of the pastry lining with water, then place the dough circle on top. Press down with your fingers to seal.

Make a pleated lid from a double layer of baking parchment and press the paper over the basin edge. Secure around the top with string, cover with foil then tie more string around the basin and over the top to make a handle. Set a trivet in a large lidded saucepan and half fill with water. Lower the basin in so that the water comes halfway up the basin. Cover the pan and steam the pudding on the hob/stovetop for 3 hours. Once cooked, lift the basin out with the string handle. Cool for a few minutes. To serve, slide a knife around the edge to loosen the pudding, place a serving plate on top of the basin and carefully invert onto the plate.

for the batter

65 g/½ cup gluten-free plain/
all-purpose flour

50 g/3½ tablespoons butter

2 large eggs, beaten

for the toad

2 gluten-free sausages

1 small dessert apple

1 small onion

60–80 ml/¼–scant ⅓ cup olive oil

sea salt and freshly ground black
pepper

a 4-hole Yorkshire pudding pan

*a piping pastry bag fitted with a large
nozzle/tip*

serves 2

Making gluten-free toad-in-the-hole batter in the same way as a
traditional batter does not work well and tends to result in a flat
(not light and airy) pancake. But a choux pastry dough makes a
great toad-in-the-hole, and you won't know that it is gluten-free.

toad-in-the-hole

Preheat the oven to 180°C (350°F) Gas 4.

For the toad, twist each sausage in half tightly to make four mini
sausages. Cut the apple into quarters and remove the core leaving the
skins on, then cut each quarter into three slices. Peel the onion and cut
into small wedges. Put the sausages, apple slices and onion in a roasting
pan and drizzle with a little olive oil. Season, then roast in the oven for
about 20 minutes until the sausages brown. Remove from the oven, then
turn the oven temperature up to 200°C (400°F) Gas 6.

For the batter, sift the flour twice to remove any lumps. Heat the butter in
a saucepan with 150 ml/⅔ cup water until the butter is melted, then
bring to the boil. Add all of the flour quickly and remove the pan from the
heat. Beat hard with a wooden spoon until the dough forms a ball and no
longer sticks to the sides of the pan. Leave to cool for about 5 minutes.
Whisk the beaten eggs into the flour mixture, a small amount at a time,
using a balloon whisk. The mixture will form a sticky paste which holds
its shape when you lift the whisk up.

Pour a large spoonful of oil into each hole of the pudding pan, then put it
in the oven for 5 minutes until the oil gets very hot. Meanwhile, spoon
the dough into the piping/pastry bag. Pipe a large ring of dough
into the hot oil in each hole of the pan. Place a
sausage and some apple and onion slices
into the centre of each hole and return to
the oven for 25–30 minutes until the
batter has risen and is crisp and golden
brown. Serve straight away.

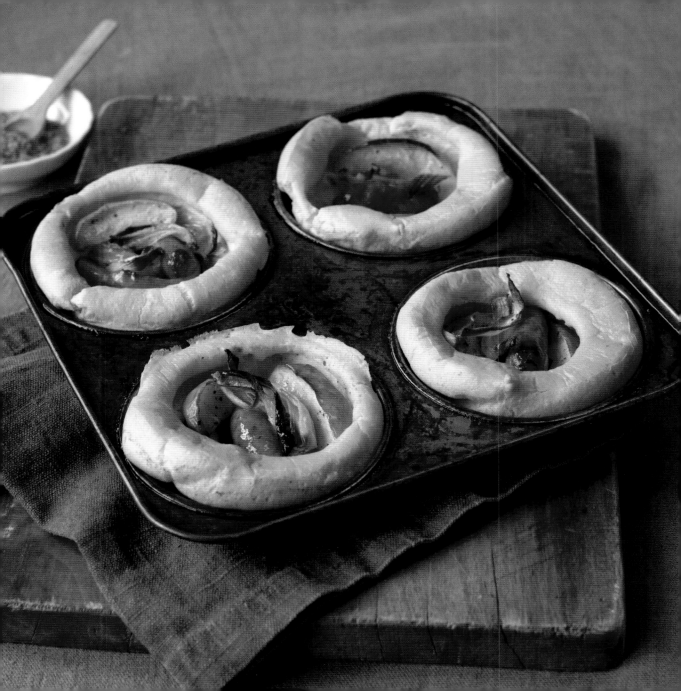

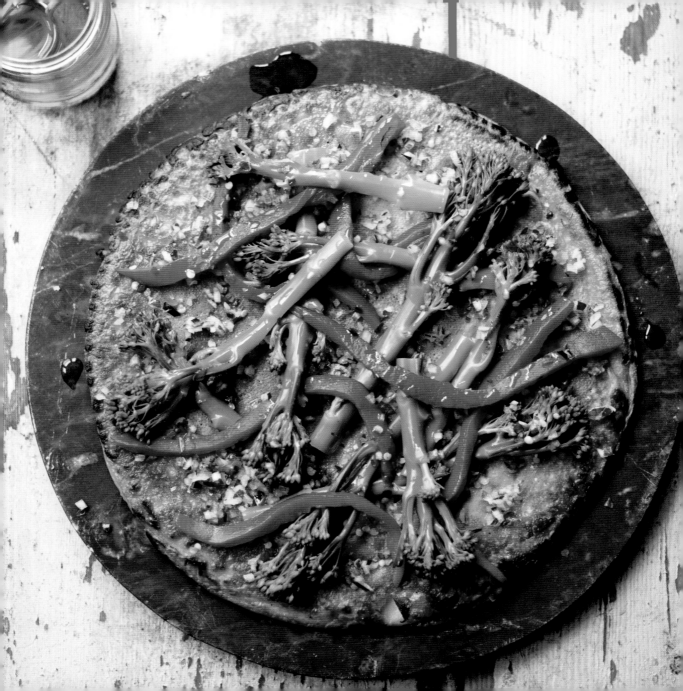

vegetarian plates

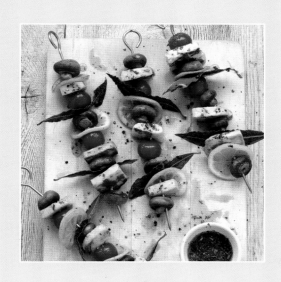

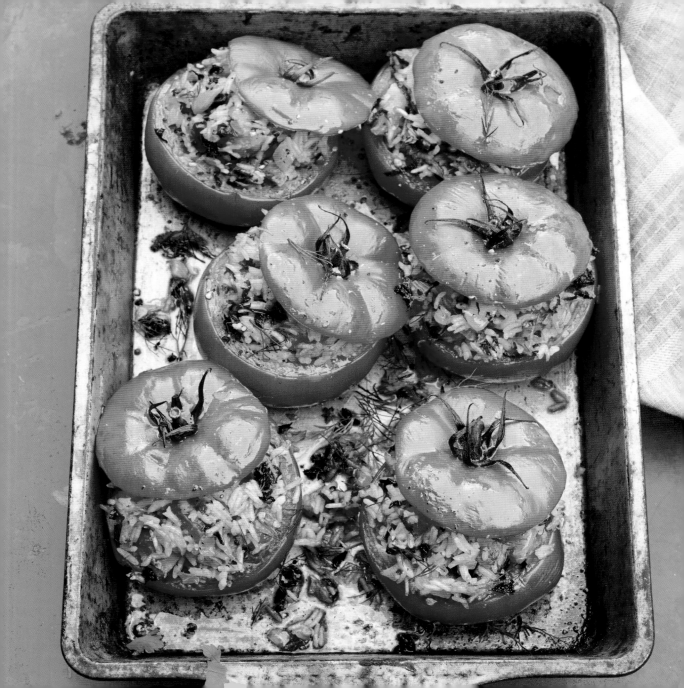

Greek rice-stuffed tomatoes

4–6 large tomatoes

3 tablespoons olive oil

1 small onion, finely chopped

150 g/¾ cup long-grain rice, rinsed

1 teaspoon tomato purée/paste

2 tablespoons freshly chopped flat-leaf parsley

2 tablespoons freshly chopped dill

2 tablespoons freshly chopped mint

1 teaspoon grated lemon zest

sea salt and freshly ground black pepper

serves 4

Evoke summer holidays on Greek islands with this Mediterranean dish, in which a few simple ingredients are transformed into a tasty and satisfying meal.

Preheat the oven to 200°C (400°F) Gas 6.

Cut the tops off the tomatoes and carefully scoop out and reserve the soft pulp. Put the tomato shells in a baking dish large enough to hold all tomatoes upright. Set aside with the caps until ready to bake.

Heat 2 tablespoons of the oil in a frying pan/skillet set over a low heat. Add the onion and fry until softened, without allowing it to brown. Add the reserved tomato pulp, the rice and tomato purée/paste. Season well with salt and pepper.

Bring the mixture to the boil and continue to cook for 10 minutes, stirring often. Stir in the parsley, dill, mint and lemon zest.

Fill the tomato shells with the rice mixture and top with their caps. Drizzle with the remaining oil, cover with foil and bake in the preheated oven for 1 hour, until the rice is tender.

Serve warm from the oven or at room temperature.

savoy cabbage ratatouille parcels

4 large leaves of savoy cabbage

1 aubergine/eggplant, sliced into 1-cm/⅜-inch rounds

2 red onions, finely diced

1 onion, finely diced

1 red (bell) pepper, deseeded and finely diced

1 yellow (bell) pepper, deseeded and finely diced

1 courgette/zucchini, finely diced

olive oil, for frying

a small bunch of fresh marjoram, to serve

for the tomato sauce

olive oil

2 garlic cloves

1 teaspoon capers

1 x 400-g/14-oz. can chopped tomatoes

1 teaspoon white sugar

sea salt

serves 4

This take on the classic Ratatouille Niçoise is designed to look extraordinary. By taking care to cook each element separately and then combining them in the parcels, the flavours are enhanced.

Preheat the oven to 160°C (325°F) Gas 3.

To make the tomato sauce, pour in enough olive oil to coat the bottom of a small saucepan and add the garlic and capers. Set over a low heat to cook them until they are just starting to turn golden brown. Add the canned tomatoes and sugar, and leave to simmer on low for 10 minutes.

Using a hand-held electric blender, purée the mixture to a smooth consistency and season with a pinch or two of salt. Pour the mixture through a fine mesh sieve/strainer into a saucepan and set aside.

Put the savoy cabbage leaves in a pan of boiling salted water and blanch for 2 minutes, then remove and pat dry with paper towels.

Preheat a frying pan/skillet over a high heat. Drizzle a little oil over the aubergine/eggplant slices, then carefully place them into the very hot pan and cook until they're just starting to blacken. Repeat on the other side, then remove and allow to cool. Dice the slices into 5-mm/¼-inch pieces.

Add a light covering of oil to a frying pan/skillet. Set over a low heat and add the onions and (bell) peppers. Cover with a generous pinch of salt and leave to cook gently until the onions are translucent – this may take about 3–5 minutes. Add the courgette/zucchini and cook for another couple of minutes stirring gently. Remove from the heat, add the aubergine/eggplant pieces and gently stir to make the ratatouille.

Place the savoy cabbage leaves into large ramekins, allowing the edges of the leaves to hang over the sides. Fill with the ratatouille mixture and fold the edges over to seal. Cover the top with foil to hold everything together.

Bake the parcels in the preheated oven for 20 minutes. At the same time, gently heat the tomato sauce. Once cooked, carefully remove the foil and turn the parcels out onto large soup plates. Spoon the tomato sauce around the edge. Garnish with the fresh marjoram and serve.

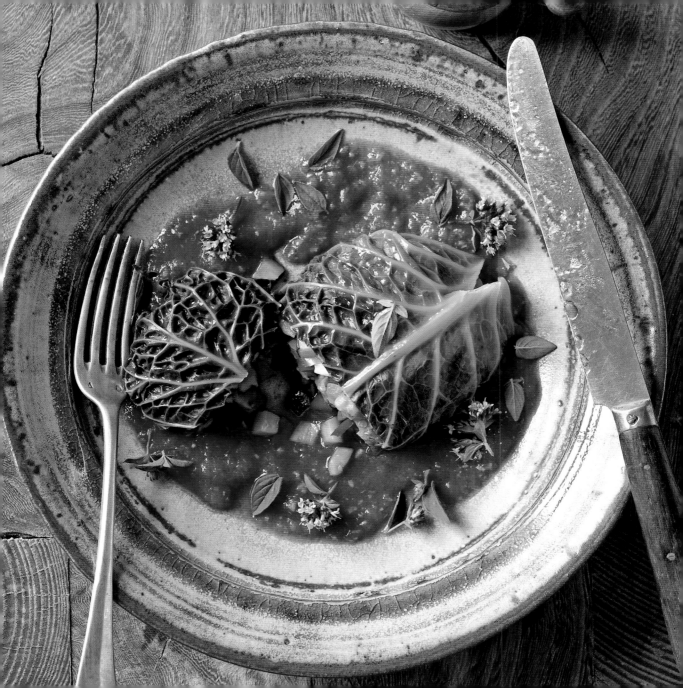

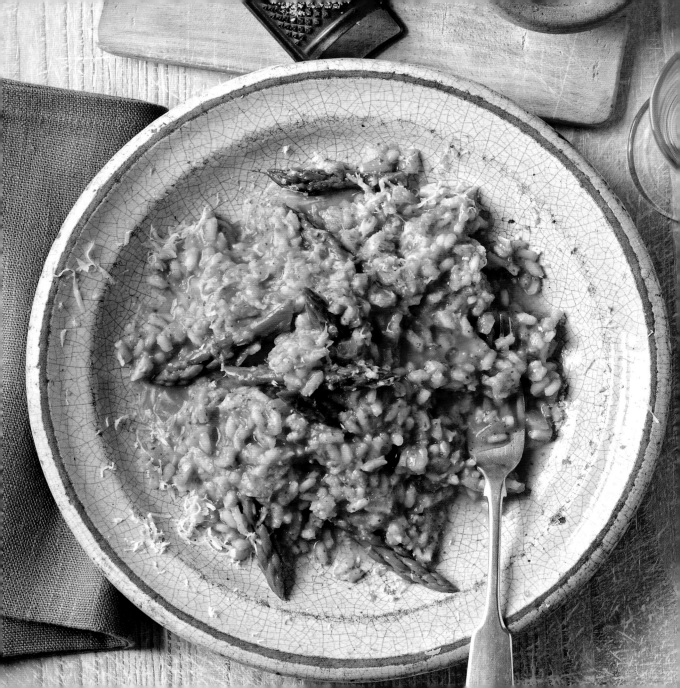

This is a great way to enjoy the wonderful flavour of asparagus, and the dramatic appearance of vibrant green in the risotto makes the dish look great, too.

asparagus risotto

4 carrots, peeled

2 celery sticks

3 brown onions

400 g/14 oz. asparagus

80 g/1¼ cups spinach leaves, washed

2 garlic cloves, thinly sliced

350 g/2 cups arborio rice

200 ml/¾ cup white wine

80 g/1¼ cups finely grated Parmesan cheese

grated zest of ½ lemon

a knob/pat of butter

sea salt

olive oil, for frying

serves 4

First, make an asparagus stock. Finely dice the carrots, celery and 2 of the onions and put in a saucepan with 1 litre/4 cups of water.

Trim about 2.5 cm/1 inch from the base of the asparagus spears and discard. Trim a further 2.5 cm/1 inch from the base of the spears, finely slice them and place in the stock water. Bring the stock to a low simmer and cook for 45 minutes. Add the spinach and simmer for 2 minutes, then blend the stock with a hand-held electric blender until smooth.

Add a little oil to a large heavy-based non-stick saucepan. Finely dice the remaining onion and add to the pan with the garlic and cook over a very low heat until just translucent. Add the rice and cook, gently stirring, until the rice is covered with oil and starts to go opaque. Add the wine and simmer until the wine is nearly all absorbed. Stirring constantly, add half of the asparagus stock and a pinch of salt and continue cooking on a low simmer until all of the stock is absorbed. Continue adding the remaining stock a little at a time until the rice is cooked and has just a little bite when tasted (there should be no excess liquid).

To finish, stir in the Parmesan cheese, lemon zest, asparagus tips and a knob/pat of butter. Serve immediately.

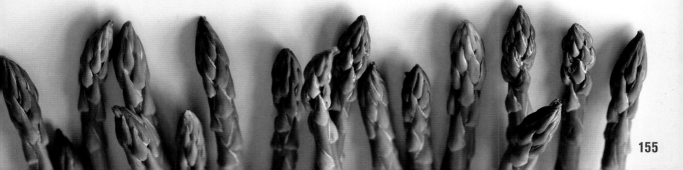

Pesto is perhaps best known when used with pasta, but it is also great when added to chicken, to salads, on top of roasted vegetables and on pizzas. This version is cheese-free. Courgettes/zucchini hold their shape well when spiralized, making them a healthy and versatile alternative to wheat pasta.

pesto 'pasta'

½–1 garlic clove, peeled, to taste

rock salt, to taste

2 handfuls of pine nuts

2 big handfuls of fresh basil, roughly chopped

extra virgin olive oil, to taste

a handful of sun-dried tomatoes, chopped

1 char-grilled red (bell) pepper, deseeded and chopped

3–4 courgettes/zucchini

sea salt and freshly ground black pepper

a spiralizer

serves 4

Using a pestle and mortar, crush the garlic with some whole rock salt. The salt helps break it down into a paste.

Warm the pine nuts in a dry frying pan/skillet set over low heat – when they are warmed they are easier to break down and release more flavour.

Add half to three-quarters of the pine nuts to the crushed garlic and set the rest aside for later. Crush to a paste. Add the basil to the mortar and grind to a paste with the pestle. Add a little pepper to taste and once you are happy with the consistency of the paste, slowly add a little olive oil. The consistency of the pesto will depend on how much oil you add and this is down to personal preference.

Add the sun-dried tomatoes, char-grilled (bell) pepper and remaining pine nuts to the pesto and stir through.

Store in the fridge in an airtight container until ready to use. The oil acts as a preservative so depending how oil-laden you made your pesto it should keep for 2 days and up to 1 week.

Spiralize the courgettes/zucchini using the spiralizer. Preheat a large frying pan/skillet with 1 tablespoon of olive oil (or a little water) over medium heat and add the courgetti. Cook for 2–3 minutes until slightly softened but still al dente. Season with salt and stir through the pesto to serve.

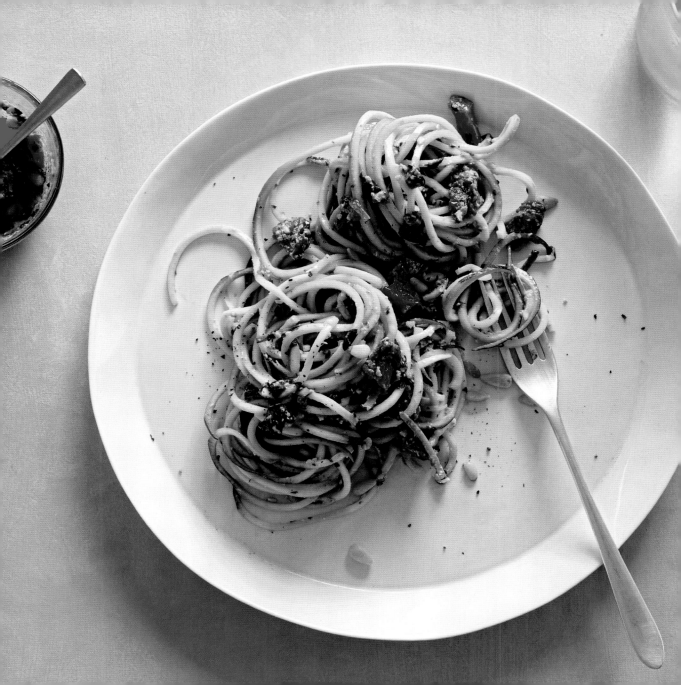

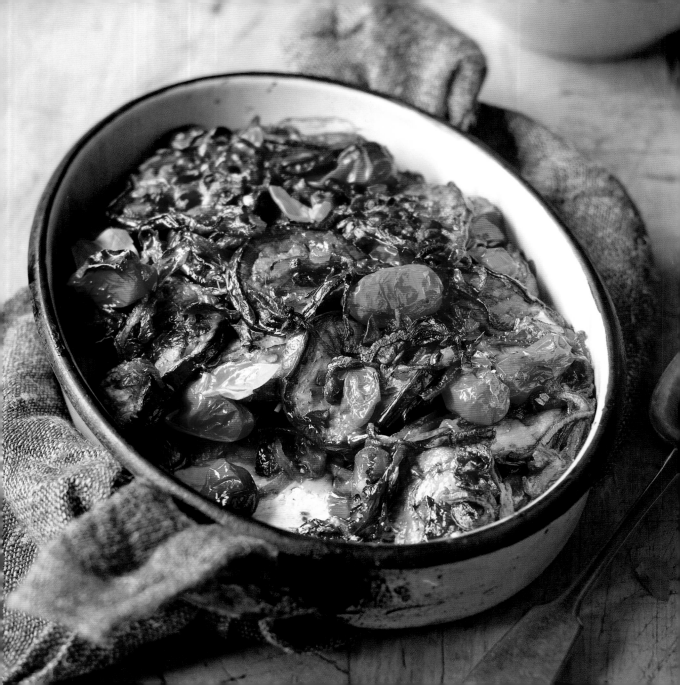

aubergine & tomato gratin

2 red onions, sliced

10 cherry tomatoes – as ripe and red as you can find

extra virgin olive oil

balsamic vinegar

3 aubergines/eggplants, topped, tailed and cut into 1-cm/½-inch slices

handful of fresh basil leaves

100 ml/6 tablespoons single/light cream

sea salt and freshly ground black pepper

serves 4-6

The velvety creaminess of this dish just screams 'bad for you', so it is such a joy to be able to scream back 'no it's not!' Aubergine/ eggplant can be quite bland if not really encouraged with good seasoning, so this is the perfect dish for them – the tomatoes, oil, non-dairy cream and herbs really bring it to life.

Preheat the oven to 200°C (400°F) Gas 6.

Toss the onions and tomatoes with some oil, salt and a drizzle of balsamic vinegar in an ovenproof dish. Roast in the preheated oven for about 15 minutes or until the skins of the tomatoes crack open and the onions are beginning to caramelize. Leave the oven on.

Meanwhile, heat a saucepan over a medium heat. Using a pastry brush, coat the aubergine/eggplant slices with oil on both sides. Fry in the hot pan until golden-brown on both sides and beginning to get soft. Transfer to a dish and give them a generous drizzle of oil. Season well with salt and a little pepper.

Layer the aubergine/eggplant slices in a casserole dish with the tomatoes, onions and basil leaves (reserving some for serving). Pour the cream over, drizzle over some oil and bake in the oven for 15–20 minutes until bubbling and golden on top.

Remove from the oven. Tear the remaining basil leaves and scatter over the top of the dish. Serve immediately.

potato bowls with mushroom, garlic, spinach & ricotta

4 large Maris Piper or other floury potatoes

a good knob/pat of butter

250 g/9 oz. button mushrooms, quartered

100 g/1 cup spinach, washed

2 garlic cloves, crushed

a splash of balsamic vinegar

200 g/7 oz. ricotta cheese

sea salt

serves 4

Jacket potatoes are the best! Here, the second cooking of the potato skins makes them extra crunchy, which offers a delicious contrast to the fluffy, whipped potato and ricotta filling.

Preheat the oven to 180°C (350°F) Gas 4.

Clean, then prick the potatoes all over with a fork, before putting them in a microwave to cook for 20 minutes on high. Remove the potatoes from the microwave and cook in the preheated oven for 45 minutes.

While the potatoes are baking, put a generous dollop of butter in a large, heavy-based frying pan/skillet and add a pinch of salt. Heat the frying pan/skillet over a medium-high heat until the butter is sizzling, then add the chopped mushrooms and cook until golden. Do not stir the mushrooms while they are cooking or they will go soggy. Turn them once when they are golden, then add the spinach, garlic and balsamic vinegar, and take off the heat. Stir together – the residual heat from the pan will cook the garlic and spinach.

Remove the potatoes and carefully, using a dry kitchen cloth or oven gloves to hold them, cut the tops off, about one-third of the way from the top. Scoop out the cooked insides of the potatoes and reserve them. Keep the oven on.

Mix the cooked mushrooms, garlic and spinach with half of the scooped-out potato flesh and half of the ricotta cheese. Fold together, before refilling the potatoes with the mixture. Cover with the remaining ricotta, crumbled over the top, and bake in the still-hot oven for 10 minutes. Serve hot.

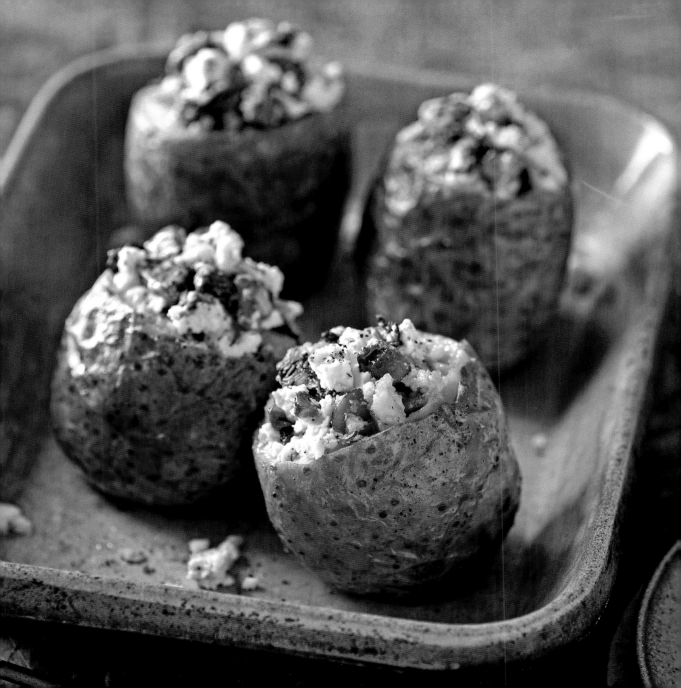

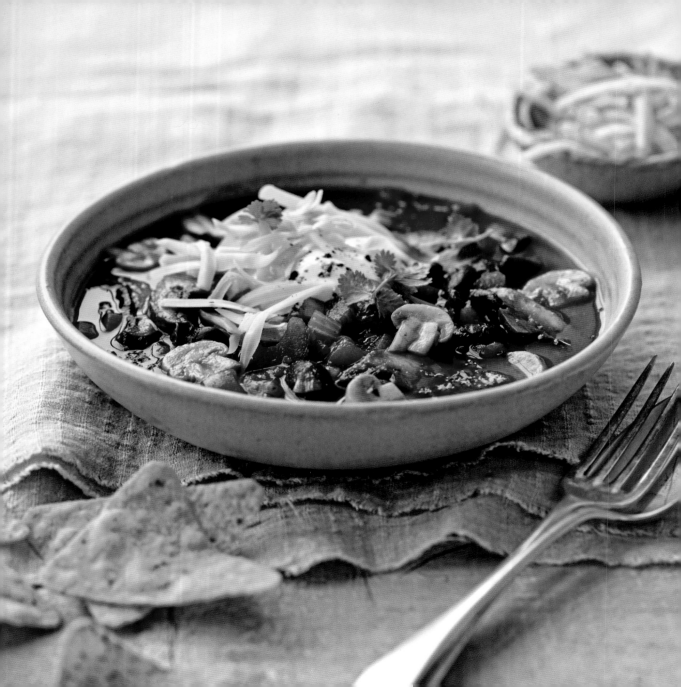

1 tablespoon olive oil

1 onion, chopped

1 garlic clove, chopped

1 celery stick, chopped

½ red (bell) pepper, deseeded and finely chopped

150 g/5 oz. field mushrooms (Portabellini), finely chopped

1 teaspoon ground cumin

a pinch of dried oregano

½ teaspoon smoked paprika

1 x 400-g/14-oz. can chopped tomatoes

1 teaspoon chipotle paste

a pinch of sugar

1 x 400-g/14-oz. can kidney beans in water, drained and rinsed

200 g/7 oz. button mushrooms, halved if large

sea salt and freshly ground black pepper

freshly chopped coriander/cilantro, to garnish

soured cream and grated Cheddar cheese (optional), to serve

serves 4

This spicy vegetarian take on a classic chilli/chili con carne is both simple and quick to make. It can also, usefully, be made a day in advance and kept in the fridge until needed. Serve with gluten-free tortilla crisps/chips or baked potatoes. It's especially good with tangy soured cream, which contrasts nicely with this rich tomato-based dish.

mushroom & bean chilli

Heat the oil in a casserole dish or Dutch oven over a medium heat. Add the onion, garlic, celery and red (bell) pepper and fry, stirring, for 5 minutes until softened. Add the field mushrooms (Portabellini), cumin, oregano and smoked paprika and fry, stirring, for 5 minutes.

Add the chopped tomatoes, 200 ml/1 scant cup of water, chipotle paste and sugar. Season with salt and pepper and stir well. Bring to the boil, then stir in the kidney beans and button mushrooms.

Lower the heat to medium and simmer, uncovered, for 15 minutes, stirring now and then. Portion into bowls and garnish with the chopped coriander/cilantro. Serve with soured cream and grated Cheddar cheese, if desired.

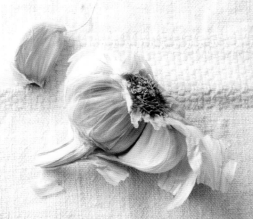

In their native Italy, farinata are nearly always cooked on a very large cast-iron pan in a searingly hot wood-fired oven, then served very simply with some black pepper.

farinata with red pepper & tender-stem broccoli

400 g/14 oz. tender-stem broccoli/ broccolini

olive oil

1 red onion, very finely chopped

small jar roasted red (bell) peppers, cut into strips

½ teaspoon dried chilli/hot red pepper flakes, or urfa chilli/chili flakes

sea salt and freshly ground black pepper

for the batter

300 g/2⅓ cups chickpea/gram flour,

1 teaspoon sea salt

2 sprigs of rosemary, leaves only, roughly chopped

extra virgin olive oil, plus regular olive oil for frying

serves 3–6

First make the batter by placing the chickpea/gram flour, salt (ground to a powder) and the rosemary leaves in a large bowl. Slowly whisk in 4 tablespoons extra virgin olive oil and 415 ml/scant 1¾ cups water, ensuring that there are no lumps. Cover and leave at room temperature for at least 4 hours (or ideally overnight).

Preheat the oven to 240°C (475°F) Gas 9. Bring a saucepan of salted water to the boil, cook the broccoli/broccolini for about 3 minutes, or until just tender. Drain, drizzle over a little olive oil and set aside. Put 2½ tablespoons of olive oil in a 24 cm/10 inch non-stick ovenproof frying pan/skillet and place on a high heat. Only when extremely hot, almost smoking, ladle on a third of the batter, which should be about 1 cm/½ inch thick, swirling around so it is evenly distributed. Leave on the high heat for exactly 1 minute, then place in the oven and cook for 5 minutes, or until it is set and the underside is crispy. Flip onto a large plate so the crispy underside is uppermost and drizzle over a very generous amount of good extra virgin olive oil. Sprinkle over some red onion, and place some red (bell) peppers and broccoli/broccolini on top. Finally sprinkle over chilli/ hot red pepper flakes and a little salt and pepper and serve.

Variation

To make an instant version of farinata, use 480 ml/2 cups sparkling/soda water instead when making the batter, as this gives the pancake a lighter texture without having to leave it to ferment. Fry in a pan/skillet as above, but instead of putting the pancake in the oven after 1 minute, turn the heat down to medium and fry for a couple of minutes until the base is set and the top is drying out, then carefully flip over and cook for another few minutes. When the pancake is cooked through, slide off and serve as above with the various toppings.

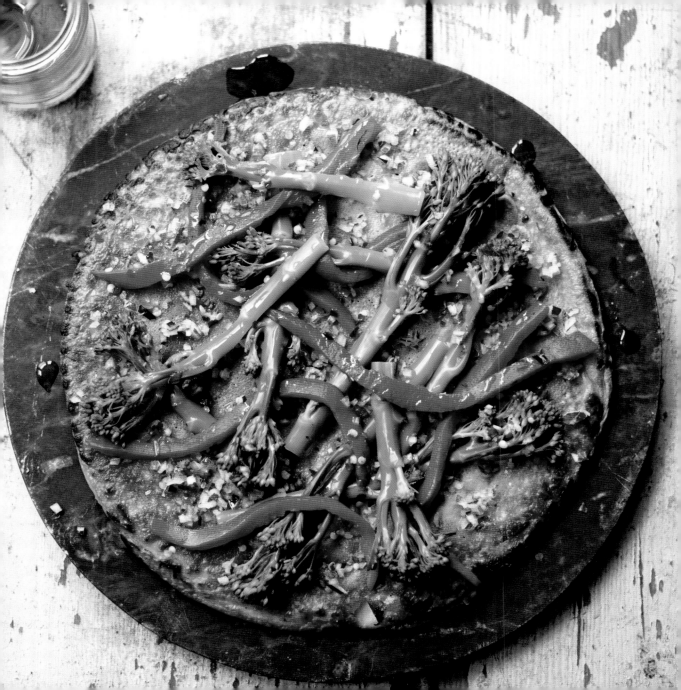

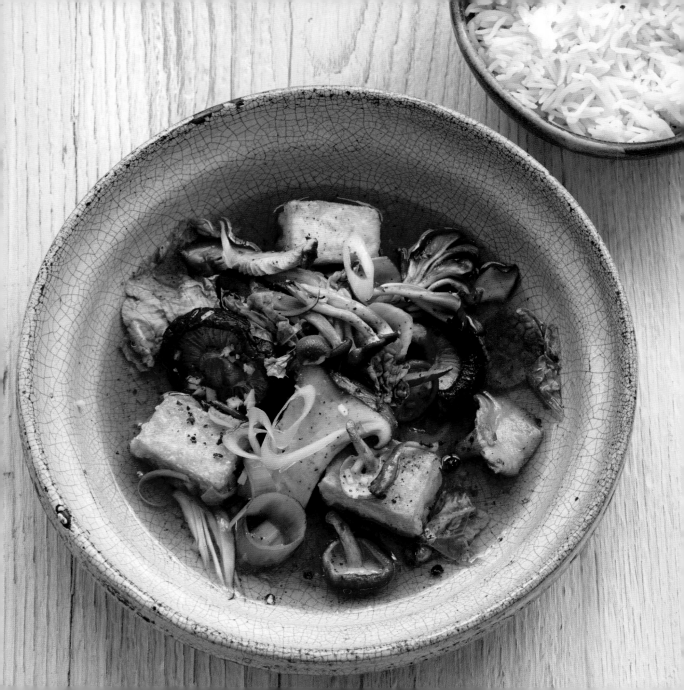

tofu & mushroom hotpot

400 g/14 oz. firm tofu, well-drained

8 dried shiitake mushrooms

1 tablespoon cornflour/cornstarch

2 tablespoons vegetable oil

½ onion, chopped

1 leek, thinly sliced

2.5-cm/1-inch piece of fresh ginger, peeled and finely chopped

1 garlic clove, chopped

¼ head of Chinese leaf/napa cabbage, roughly chopped

3 tablespoons rice wine or Amontillado sherry

a pinch of Chinese five-spice powder

150 g/5½ oz. assorted fresh mushrooms (oyster, shiitake, eryngii), large ones halved

1 tablespoon tamari

a pinch of sugar

1 teaspoon sesame oil

sea salt

chopped spring onion/scallion, to garnish

serves 4

Mushrooms and tofu have a natural affinity, and they are combined here in a fresh vegetarian take on a classic Chinese hotpot. Serve with steamed rice or boiled gluten-free noodles.

Wrap the tofu in paper towels and place a weighty item (such as a heavy baking sheet) on top. Leave for at least 10 minutes to let the excess moisture drain.

Soak the dried shiitake mushrooms in 200 ml/1 scant cup of hot water for 20 minutes. Strain through a fine-mesh sieve/strainer, reserving the soaking liquid. Trim and discard the tough stalks from the shiitake and cut them in half.

Cut the tofu into cubes and roll them in the cornflour/cornstarch to coat. Heat 1 tablespoon of the oil in a frying pan/skillet. Fry the tofu for 5 minutes over a medium-high heat, turning over during frying, until lightly browned on all sides.

Heat the remaining oil in a casserole dish or Dutch oven over a medium heat. Add the onion, leek, ginger and garlic and fry, stirring, for 2 minutes. Add the Chinese leaf/napa cabbage and fry for a further 2 minutes. Mix in the rice wine or sherry and five-spice powder and cook for 1 minute. Add the fried tofu, soaked shiitake and the fresh mushrooms.

Pour in the reserved shiitake soaking liquid, add the tamari and the pinch of sugar. Bring to the boil. Cover and cook over a medium heat for 15 minutes. Uncover and cook for 10 minutes, stirring gently now and then. Season with salt. Stir in the sesame oil. Serve straight away, garnished with chopped spring onion/scallion.

polenta with wild mushrooms

400 g/14 oz. assorted mushrooms
(half cultivated, half wild)

200 g/1⅓ cups instant polenta

2 tablespoons butter

1 tablespoon olive oil

½ red onion, sliced

1 garlic clove, chopped

1 sprig of fresh rosemary

sea salt and freshly ground black
pepper

freshly chopped parsley, to garnish

grated Parmesan cheese, to serve

serves 4

**Comfort food, Italian-style! This dish features sautéed wild and
cultivated mushrooms on a bed of polenta. Simple but delizioso!**

Cut the cultivated mushrooms into 1-cm/½-inch-thick slices. Trim the
wild mushrooms.

Bring 2 litres/quarts of generously salted water to the boil in a large
saucepan. Add the polenta in a steady stream, stirring vigorously with
a wooden spoon as you do so in order to prevent lumps from forming.
Cook, stirring, until the mixture thickens, a matter of around 5 minutes.
Mix in the butter and keep warm over a low heat.

Heat the olive oil in a large, heavy-bottomed frying pan/skillet. Add the
red onion, garlic and rosemary and fry for 2 minutes, until the onion has
softened. Add the wild and cultivated mushrooms and fry over a high
heat for 3–4 minutes, until browned and just softened. Season with salt
and freshly ground black pepper. Discard the rosemary sprig.

Serve the warm polenta topped with the mushroom mixture and plenty of
extra black pepper. Garnish with chopped parsley, and serve with grated
Parmesan cheese on the side.

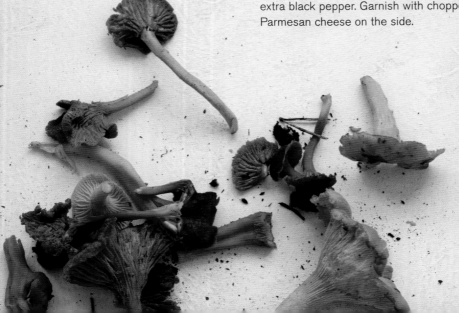

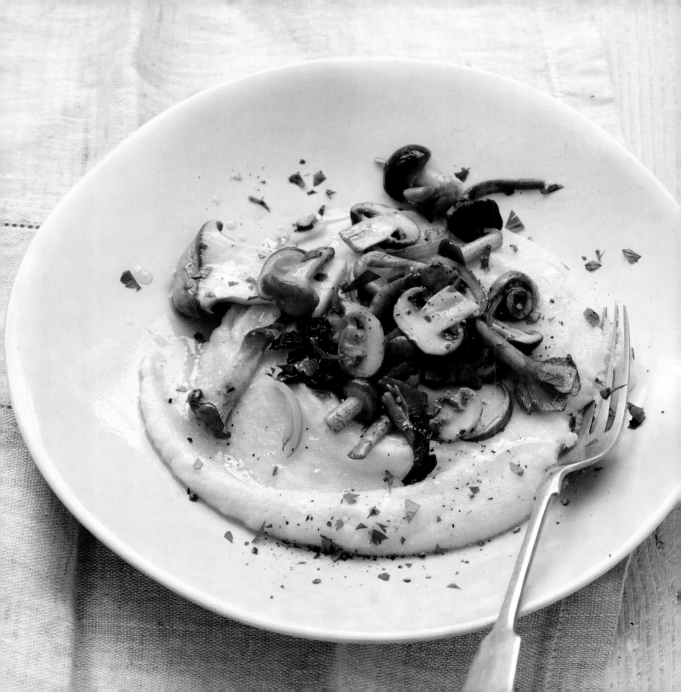

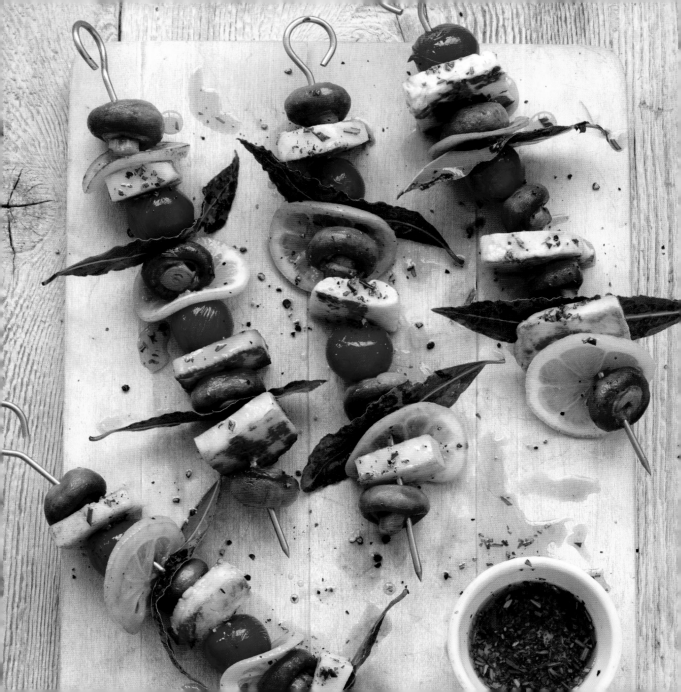

250 g/9 oz. halloumi cheese, cut into 16 even-sized pieces

16 even-sized button mushrooms, stalks trimmed off

12 cherry tomatoes

2 tablespoons olive oil

1 tablespoon freshly chopped parsley leaves

8 fresh bay leaves

8 thin lemon slices

sea salt and freshly ground black pepper

8 metal cooking skewers

serves 4

With their natural bouncy texture, mushrooms lend themselves to being grilled/broiled or barbecued. Pleasingly plump button mushrooms, salty halloumi cheese and juicy cherry tomatoes combine well, offering a taste of the Mediterranean. Cook over a barbecue for extra flavour. Serve with a rocket/arugula, cucumber and tomato salad.

mushroom & halloumi kebabs

Preheat the grill/broiler.

In a large bowl, toss together the halloumi cheese, button mushrooms, cherry tomatoes, olive oil and parsley. Season with salt and pepper, bearing in mind the natural saltiness of the halloumi.

Thread the cheese, mushrooms, cherry tomatoes, bay leaves and lemon slices onto the eight skewers.

Grill/broil the halloumi skewers for 5 minutes, turning over halfway through, until the halloumi is golden-brown. Serve at once.

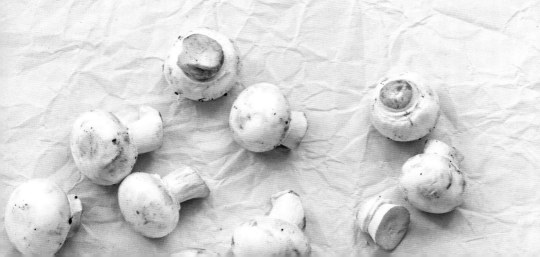

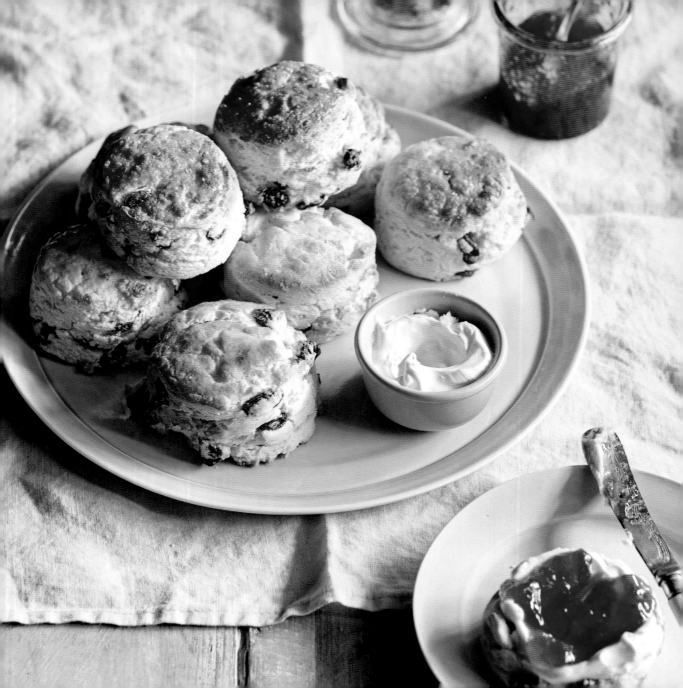

baking

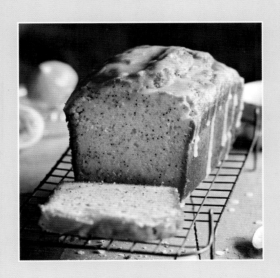

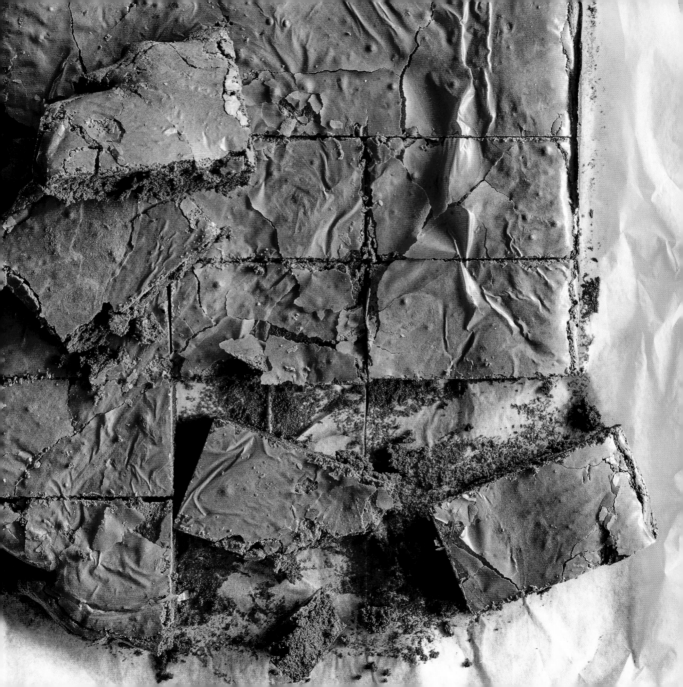

These brownies are delicious served warm with ice cream or custard. You can vary them by adding pecans, white chocolate chips, fresh raspberries or dried cranberries into the batter.

brownies

250 g/9 oz. dark/bittersweet chocolate, chips or chopped

125 g/1 stick unsalted butter

125 g/1 stick salted butter

120 g/¾ cup plus 1 tablespoon plain/all-purpose gluten-free flour

60 g/½ cup cocoa powder

5 eggs

175 g/¾ cup plus 2 tablespoons soft light brown sugar

200 g/1 cup caster/granulated sugar

a large square baking pan greased and lined with baking parchment (about 38 x 28 cm/15 x 11 inches)

makes 12–16

Preheat the oven to 190°C (375°F) Gas 5.

Either in a jug/pitcher in bursts of 10 seconds in the microwave, or in a heatproof bowl set over a pan of simmering water, melt the chocolate and butters together. Stir to combine until molten and smooth, and then cool slightly.

Tip the flour and cocoa powder into a large mixing bowl.

In another large bowl, or the bowl of a free-standing mixer, combine the eggs and both sugars. Either by hand or with the whisk attachment of the mixer, whisk up the eggs and sugar vigorously until thick and pale. Once pale and thick, continue to mix the eggs on a slow speed and pour in the melted chocolate and butter mixture. When these are fully combined, stop whisking and add the flour and cocoa mixture. (You need to stop the whisk at this stage to avoid a flour shower.)

Whisk again, beginning slowly and briefly increasing the speed once combined. Within a minute there should be no lumps remaining and you'll have a thick, glossy, chocolatey batter. Pour the batter into the prepared baking pan and level with a spoon or spatula. Bake in the preheated oven for 25 minutes, checking after 20 minutes, until risen with a papery crust. The top of the brownie may crack, but don't worry, it will sink back together on cooling.

Remove the pan from the oven and gently shake the brownie or press the top with your finger. It should feel almost set, but with a slight wobble.

Set the pan on a wire rack and cool for as long as you can resist before portioning into 16 sensible or 12 generous pieces. (This brownie portions like a dream if placed in the fridge for a couple of hours first.)

Enjoy right away or store in an airtight container in the fridge for up to 1 week and warm up before serving.

Everybody has an opinion on what should or shouldn't be in a rocky road: cherries, sultanas/golden raisins, nuts? Why not ring the changes regularly trying the variations below. As it's a no-bake recipe, it's perfect for little ones to help out with.

rocky road

150 g/5 oz. dark/bittersweet chocolate, chopped

75 g/5 tablespoons unsalted butter, cubed

50 g/3 tablespoons golden syrup/light corn syrup

150 g/5 oz. gluten-free digestive biscuits/graham crackers

50 g/⅓ cup blanched almonds, chopped

75 g/½ cup glacé/candied cherries, halved

100 g/2½ cups mini marshmallows

gluten-free icing/confectioners' sugar, for dusting (optional)

a 20-cm/8-inch square baking pan lined with baking parchment

makes 12–16

In a saucepan, gently melt together the chocolate, butter and golden syrup/light corn syrup until completely combined. Remove from the heat and set aside.

Break up the digestive biscuits/graham crackers into a rough rubble – you can chop them or put them in a plastic food bag, wrap in a kitchen cloth and bash with a rolling pin. Put the biscuit bits into a large bowl and stir in the almonds, cherries and mini marshmallows. Pour over the melted chocolate mixture and stir together with a large spoon or spatula until everything is well coated.

Tip the mixture into the prepared baking pan, spreading out and lightly pressing down. Put the pan in the fridge and allow to set for 3–4 hours until firm.

Invert the pan onto a chopping board to remove the rocky road. Peel off the baking parchment, then slice into 12–16 pieces.

Dust with icing/confectioners' sugar before serving, if you like. Store in an airtight container for up to 1 week.

Variations
To make things a bit more grown-up, swap the cherries for 50 g/⅓ cup chopped crystallized ginger and add 75 g/⅔ cup dark/bittersweet chocolate chunks; or at Christmas time you can throw in 50 g/⅓ cup dried cranberries and the zest of 1 large orange.

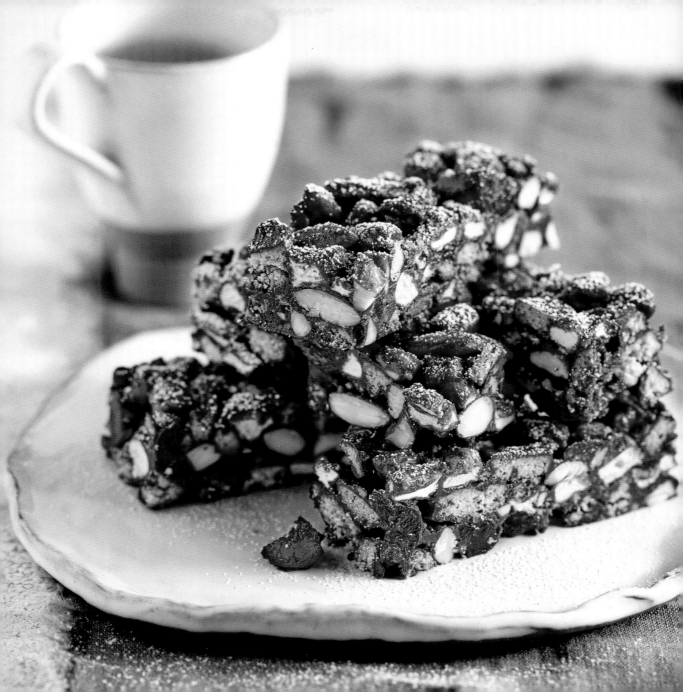

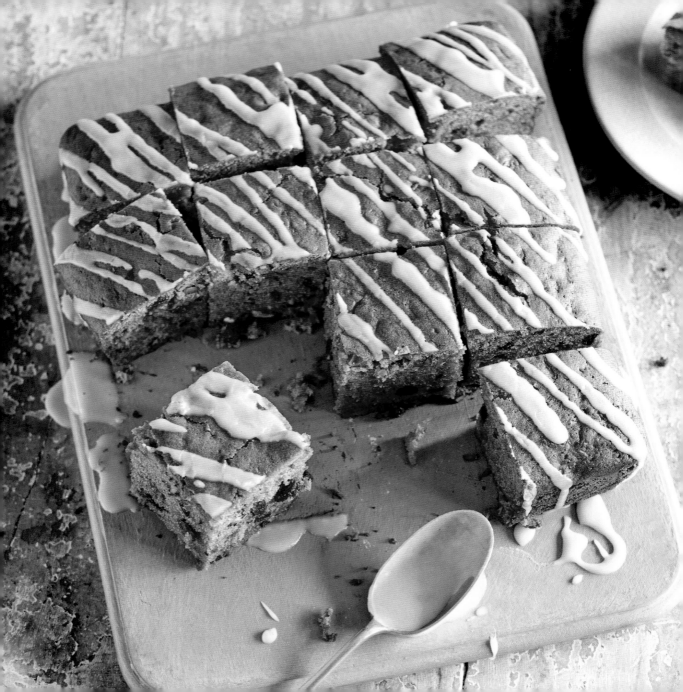

carrot cake

240 g/1¼ cups soft light brown sugar

250 ml/1 cup sunflower oil

4 eggs

270 g/1¾ cups plain/all-purpose gluten-free flour

1 tablespoon gluten-free baking powder

½ teaspoon xanthan gum

½ teaspoon salt

1 teaspoon bicarbonate of soda/baking soda

2 teaspoons mixed spice/apple pie spice

200 g/1 medium carrot, grated

grated zest of 1 orange

100 g/⅔ cup sultanas/golden raisins

75 g/½ cup pecan nuts, chopped

for the orange glaze

150 g/1⅓ cups gluten-free icing/confectioners' sugar

3–5 tablespoons freshly squeezed orange juice

a 20-cm/8-inch square cake pan greased and lined with baking parchment

serves 12

A good carrot cake is essential ammunition in any baker's arsenal. It can be spruced up with cream-cheese frosting for special occasions, drizzled with orange glaze to keep it dairy-free or left naked for easy transportation on picnics. It's a doddle to make, with only very slight exertion required in the form of grating carrots. This recipe contains both nuts and sultanas/golden raisins, but will work without them, if that's your preference. It's also worth noting that should you find yourself with a glut of parsnips, simply substitute these for the carrots — the result will be different, but every bit as tasty.

Preheat the oven to 170°C (325°F) Gas 3.

To a large bowl, or the bowl of a free-standing mixer, add the sugar, oil and eggs. Whisk on a medium-high speed until thickened and slightly pale. Add the flour, baking powder, xanthan gum, salt, bicarbonate of soda/baking soda and mixed spice/apple pie spice to the bowl and whisk again until you have a smooth, thick batter. Add the grated carrot, orange zest, sultanas/golden raisins and pecan nuts, and stir in until well combined.

Spoon or pour the mixture into the cake pan and bake in the preheated oven for 45–55 minutes, checking the cake after 45 minutes. The cake is done when it's risen and springs back when pressed lightly on the top — a skewer inserted into the centre of the cake should come out without any wet batter clinging to it.

Place the pan onto a wire rack and allow to cool completely. Once cooled, gently remove from the pan, loosening with a knife if necessary.

At this stage the cake can be dusted with icing/confectioners' sugar and served just as it is. For a dairy-free adornment, as pictured, prepare the orange glaze. Sift the icing/confectioners' sugar into a bowl. Stir in the orange juice a tablespoon at a time and mix well to form a viscous paste. Drizzle over the cake and allow to set before serving.

lemon poppy seed drizzle loaf

Loaf cakes are lovely to have around. They slice well and their smaller size and simplicity means they are the perfect option for those 'just because' days when a bake seems essential, but there's no particular celebration in the offing. If you don't like poppy seeds, or don't have them to hand, you can leave them out.

240 ml/1 cup whole milk

15 g/1 tablespoon sunflower oil

2 eggs

260 g/1¾ cups plain/all-purpose gluten-free flour

3½ teaspoons gluten-free baking powder

¼ teaspoon salt

⅜ teaspoon xanthan gum

250 g/1¼ cups caster/granulated sugar

grated zest of 2 lemons

75 g/5 tablespoons unsalted butter, softened

2 tablespoons poppy seeds

crème fraîche, to serve

for the glaze

freshly squeezed juice of 2 lemons

100 g/½ cup caster/granulated sugar

a 900-g/2-lb. loaf pan, greased and lined with baking parchment

serves 8–10

Preheat the oven to 180°C (350°F) Gas 4.

In a jug/pitcher, combine the milk, oil and eggs.

To a large bowl, or the bowl of a free-standing mixer, add the flour, baking powder, salt, xanthan gum, sugar, lemon zest and softened butter. Using either a hand-held electric whisk or a free-standing mixer, slowly mix the dry ingredients and the butter until they resemble fine breadcrumbs. Continue to mix on a slow speed and pour in the wet ingredients. Once combined, turn the speed to medium and mix for 3–5 minutes until the batter thickens. Add the poppy seeds and mix until evenly distributed. Pour or spoon the batter into the loaf pan and level with the back of a spatula.

Bake in the preheated oven for 40–45 minutes until it is risen, golden and springs back when pressed lightly on the top. Remove from the oven and check that it is baked by inserting a clean skewer into the centre of the cake. It should come out clean or crumbed with no wet batter clinging to it.

Put the pan onto a wire rack and allow to rest for 1–2 minutes while you mix together the glaze.

Stir together the lemon juice and sugar in a bowl.

Without removing the cake from the pan, prick the surface all over with a fork or skewer, then pour over the glaze – it's important to do this while the cake is still warm. Leave the cake to cool completely in the pan on the wire rack, by which time the glaze will have crystallized and set.

Remove the loaf from the pan, loosening the edges with a palette or table knife if necessary. Slice and serve, with a dollop of crème fraîche, if liked.

Try this with other citrus fruits, too – both oranges and limes work well.

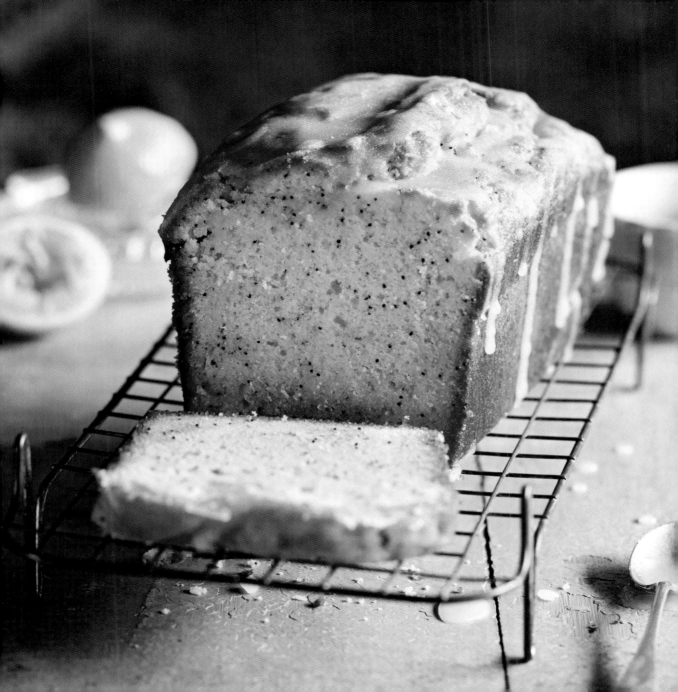

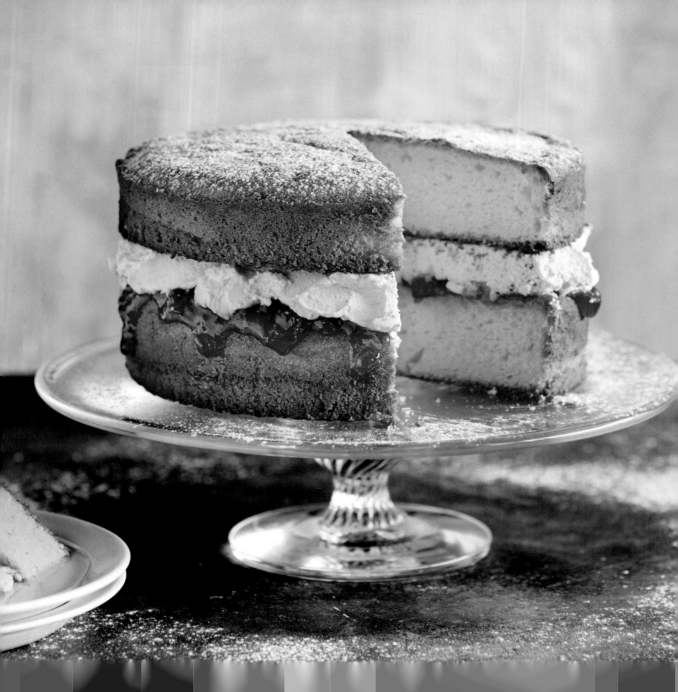

360 ml/1½ cups whole milk

1½ tablespoons sunflower oil

1 teaspoon vanilla extract

3 eggs

390 g/2⅔ cups plain/all-purpose gluten-free flour

5 teaspoons gluten-free baking powder

½ teaspoon salt

½ teaspoon xanthan gum

375 g/1¾ cups plus 2 tablespoons caster/granulated sugar

105 g/7 tablespoons unsalted butter, softened

for the filling

150 ml/⅔ cup double/heavy cream

1 tablespoon gluten-free icing/confectioners' sugar, plus extra for dusting

2 tablespoons cornflour/cornstarch

100 g/scant ½ cup strawberry jam/jelly

caster/granulated sugar, for dusting (optional)

2 x 20-cm/8-inch round cake pans, greased and lined with baking parchment

serves 12

This cake is simple but stunning – the combination of textures and flavours just works. Traditional it is, but if it ain't broke...

Victoria sponge cake

Preheat the oven to 180°C (350°F) Gas 4.

In a jug/pitcher, combine the milk, oil, vanilla extract and eggs.

To a large bowl, or the bowl of a free-standing mixer, add the flour, baking powder, salt, xanthan gum, sugar and softened butter. Using either a hand-held electric whisk or a free-standing mixer, slowly mix until the mixture resembles fine breadcrumbs. Continue to mix on a slow speed and pour in the wet ingredients. Once combined, turn the speed to medium and mix for 3–5 minutes until the batter thickens. Divide the mixture evenly between the pans and level with a spoon or spatula.

Bake the cakes in the preheated oven for 40–45 minutes until they are risen, golden and spring back when pressed lightly on the top.

Remove from the oven and check that the cakes are baked by inserting a clean skewer into the centre of each cake. It should come out clean or crumbed but without any wet batter clinging to it.

Put the pans onto a wire rack and allow to cool completely.

Once cooled, gently remove from the pans, loosening the edges with a table knife if necessary, and level the bottom layer if required.

Stabilize the cream for the filling by whisking together the double/heavy cream, icing/confectioners' sugar and cornflour/cornstarch in a bowl. Watch the cream like a hawk as it whisks; it can quickly become overworked. You are aiming for fluffy peaks that are just stiff enough to support the top cake layer when assembled.

Place the first layer of sponge onto a serving plate or stand and top with strawberry jam/jelly. Follow with a healthy layer of whipped cream. Place the top layer on top and generously dust with icing/confectioners' sugar, or caster/granulated sugar for a more traditional finish. Serve in slices.

60 g/½ cup raisins

1 tablespoon rum

300 g/2⅓ cups chestnut flour

¼ teaspoon fine sea salt

¼ teaspoon bourbon vanilla powder

grated zest of 1 orange

50 g/¼ cup olive oil

450–625 ml/2–3 cups rice milk

60 g/⅓ cup pine nuts

60 g/⅓ cup chopped hazelnuts

leaves pulled from 1 fresh rosemary sprig

whipped gluten-free soy cream or agave syrup, to serve

24-cm/9½-in. springform cake pan, well oiled

serves 8

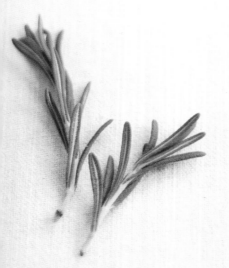

Castagnaccio, or chestnut cake, is a traditional Tuscan dessert and one of the few Italian desserts that doesn't require a lot of sugar and eggs. This vegan cake is something in between sweet and savoury; the chestnut flour gives it a mild sweet taste but since no other sweetener is used, it's not very sweet. However, it's still wonderfully simple and tasty – once a poor man's dessert, it's now a delicacy enjoyed by gourmets everywhere.

castagnaccio

Soak the raisins in a bowl with the rum and 2 tablespoons hot water while you prepare the other ingredients.

Preheat the oven to 200°C (400°F) Gas 6.

Sift together the flour, salt and vanilla powder in a bowl, then mix in the orange zest and half of the oil. Slowly whisk in the milk, adding just enough to get a smooth, soft batter; it should be soft enough to fall from the whisk, but not too liquid.

Drain the soaked raisins and pat them dry, then add them to the cake mixture.

Pour the mixture into the prepared cake pan until about 2 cm/¾ inch thick in the pan – shallower is fine but deeper could result in a soggy texture. Sprinkle the pine nuts, hazelnuts and rosemary leaves evenly over the top of the cake and press them in lightly. Drizzle the remaining olive oil over the top.

Bake in the preheated oven for 30–40 minutes, or until a thin, cracked crust has formed. The inside should still be soft and moist. Allow to cool completely in the pan before removing to serve.

Serve the cake with a dollop of whipped soy cream or a drizzle of agave syrup. It will keep for a couple of days in an airtight container.

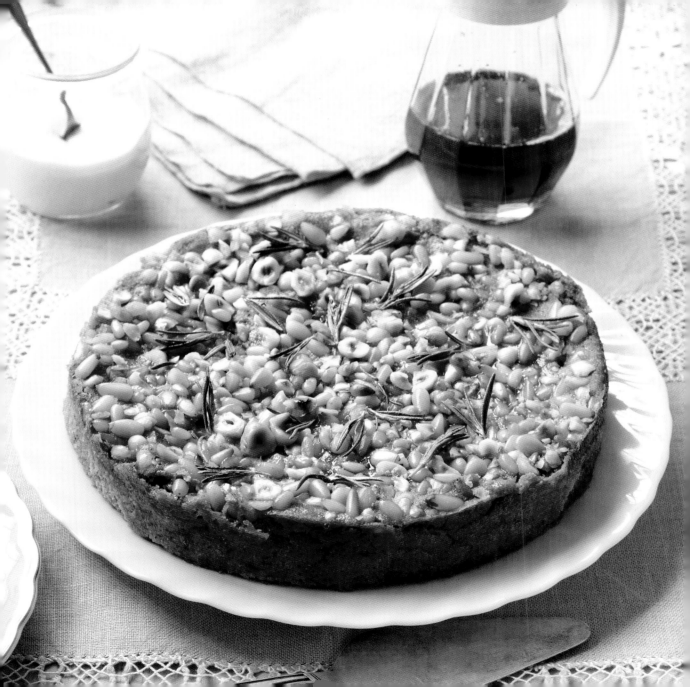

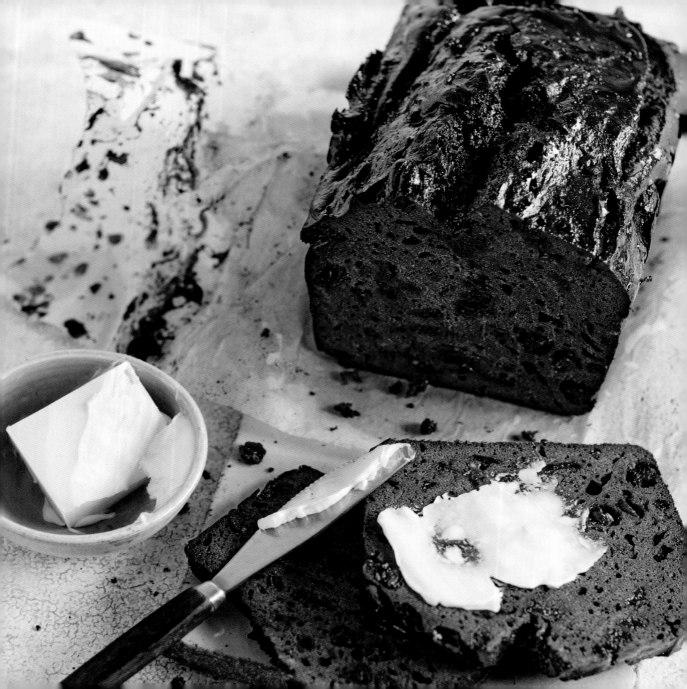

'malt' loaf

This is not technically a malt loaf, as traditional malt extract is made from barley, but the recipe uses brown teff flour and molasses to impart a similar flavour. Laden with dried fruit, it feels almost nutritious enough for a quick breakfast, or you can slice and serve with lashings of slightly salted butter and a cup of tea for an afternoon pick-me-up. The loaf can be served as soon as it's cool enough, but ideally, wrap and keep for 24–48 hours before slicing, to allow the stickiness to intensify.

150 g/1 cup chopped dried dates

220 ml/scant 1 cup hot black tea, made with 2 tea bags

100 ml/6½ tablespoons black treacle/molasses, plus extra for brushing

50 g/¼ cup soft light brown sugar

115 g/¾ cup brown teff flour

115 g/¾ cup plain/all-purpose gluten-free flour

1 teaspoon gluten-free baking powder

½ teaspoon xanthan gum

¼ teaspoon fine sea salt

15 g/1 tablespoon sunflower oil

2 eggs

175 g/1 generous cup sultanas/golden raisins

butter, softened, to serve (optional)

a 900-g/2-lb. loaf pan greased and lined with baking parchment

serves 8–10

Preheat the oven to 170°C (325°F) Gas 3.

Put the dates and tea into a saucepan and bring to a simmer over a gentle heat for 5 minutes until the dates have softened.

Remove from the heat and, using a stick blender, blitz until almost smooth, about 30 seconds–1 minute. If you don't have a stick blender, allow the dates to simmer for a further 5–10 minutes, remove from the heat and continue without blending them.

Stir in the treacle/molasses and brown sugar until well combined, then add the flours, baking powder, xanthan gum, salt, oil and eggs. Beat with a wooden spoon until smooth – the batter will be quite thick!

Stir in the sultanas/golden raisins, then transfer the mixture to the prepared loaf pan. Level and bake in the preheated oven for 1 hour, checking after 50 minutes that the top of the loaf isn't browning too much. Cover with foil if it is.

Take the loaf out of the oven once it feels firm and allow to cool in the pan. Brush the top of the cake with extra treacle/molasses while still warm. Remove the loaf from the pan when cool and, ideally, wrap in baking parchment and foil. Allow to rest for a day or two before eating.

Malt loaf should be served with softened butter to spread onto slices at the table and can be sliced and lightly toasted to serve warm, if desired, or to bring it back to life if it has become a little stale.

225 g/8 oz. whole fresh cherries, halved and stoned/pitted

50 g/⅓ cup sour/tart cherries, roughly chopped

flaked/slivered almonds, to sprinkle

unsweetened cocoa powder, to dust (optional)

for the cherry syrup

600 ml/2½ cups cherry juice

clear honey (or maple syrup), to taste (optional)

for the pastry

80 g/⅔ cup arrowroot

185 g/generous 1¾ cups almond flour

80 g/5½ tablespoons coconut butter

1 egg, plus 1 beaten egg, for brushing

for the almond frangipane

270 g/2¾ cups ground almonds

150 g/generous ½ cup clear honey

75 ml/scant ⅓ cup milk

3 tablespoons coconut flour

seeds from 1 vanilla pod/bean

2½ teaspoons pure almond extract

3 eggs

a 30 x 25-cm/12 x 10-inch baking pan, greased and lined with baking parchment

serves 8–10

frangipane tray bake

Enjoy a slice of this tray bake as a dessert or with a selection of other afternoon tea treats. It is delicious served with crème anglaise spiced with cardamom pods. You can also try making it with different fruit toppings – a rhubarb frangipane tray bake is the next best choice following cherry.

To make the cherry syrup, pour the cherry juice into a saucepan and simmer over a medium heat until the juice reduces down and is thick and glossy. You can add a little honey or maple syrup if the result is too sharp for your taste. Set aside until ready to serve.

Preheat the oven to 180°C (350°F) Gas 4.

To make the pastry, mix together the arrowroot and almond flour in a large mixing bowl and rub in the coconut butter.

In a separate bowl, beat the egg and 3–4 tablespoons of water together and add this to the flour mixture. Mix together and form a dough. Roll out between two pieces of clingfilm/plastic wrap to the size of the baking pan and transfer to the pan, removing the clingfilm/plastic wrap.

Brush the pastry with the beaten egg and bake in the preheated oven for 10 minutes, or until golden. Keep the oven on.

To make the almond frangipane, mix all of the ingredients together.

Spread the almond frangipane evenly across the baked pastry base and top with the halved and sour/tart cherries. Sprinkle with flaked/slivered almonds and bake in the still hot oven for 20–30 minutes until golden.

Drizzle with the reserved cherry syrup and dust with cocoa powder if desired, then slice and serve.

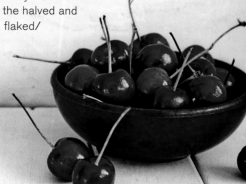

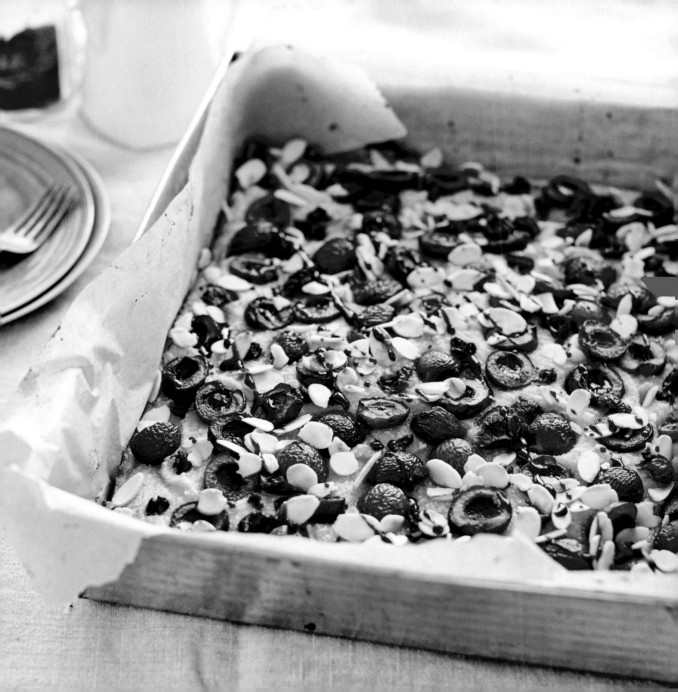

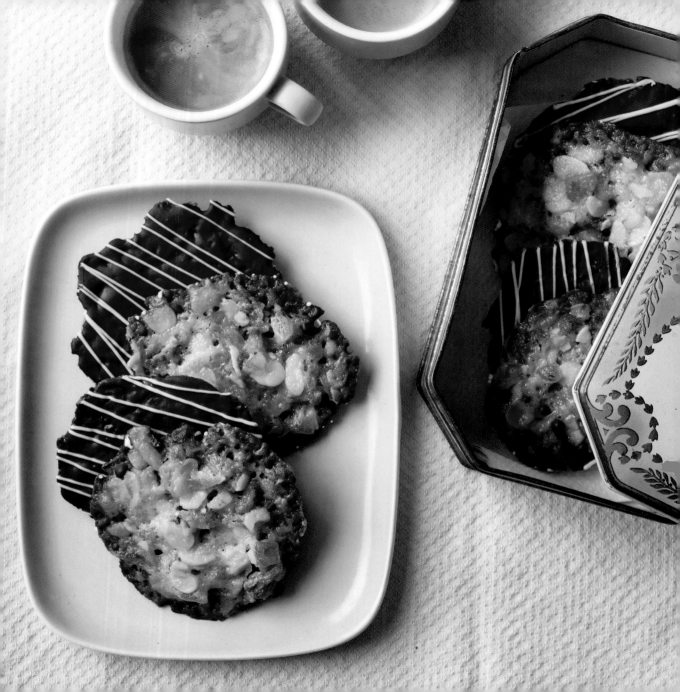

These delicious, delicate little Florentines make great petits fours – although they're equally nice with a morning brew. If you're in a hurry, serve them with a simple zigzag of white chocolate drizzled over the top to decorate. For something a little more luxurious, first coat the bases with really good-quality dark/bittersweet chocolate, and then drizzle the white on top of that.

candied pineapple & stem ginger florentines

60 g/4 tablespoons butter

60 g/⅓ cup caster/granulated sugar

1 tablespoon clear honey

a pinch of fine sea salt

50 g/⅓ cup plus 1 tablespoon plain/all-purpose gluten-free flour

50 g/⅓ cup flaked/slivered almonds

50 g/⅓ cup candied pineapple, chopped

50 g/1½ oz. stem ginger, chopped

1 tablespoon double/heavy cream

200 g/7 oz. dark/bittersweet chocolate, broken into pieces (optional)

50 g/1½ oz. white chocolate

2 baking sheets lined with baking parchment

makes about 15

Preheat the oven to 180°C (350°F) Gas 4.

Melt the butter, sugar and honey together in a small saucepan set over a low heat. Remove from the heat and leave to cool slightly. Stir in all the remaining ingredients, except the chocolates.

Drop teaspoonfuls of the mixture onto the prepared baking sheets, leaving a little space for spreading between each one.

Bake in the preheated oven for 8–10 minutes, until golden.

Remove from the oven, leave to cool slightly and then transfer to a wire rack.

Put the dark/bittersweet chocolate (if using) and white chocolate, into separate heatproof bowls and set each over a saucepan of barely simmering water to melt. Decorate the Florentine tops with a zigzag of melted chocolate if using just white chocolate. If using both, spread the smoother side of each Florentine with melted dark/bittersweet chocolate, and leave to set, then decorate the set chocolate with a zigzag of melted white chocolate.

Store in an airtight container in a cool place (but not the fridge), so the chocolate doesn't melt, and eat within 3 days.

Scones are tricky to master in gluten-free form since gluten-free flour absorbs more liquid than wheat flour. But these are great!

classic scones

225 g/1½ cups plain/all-purpose gluten-free flour, plus extra for dusting

40 g/3 tablespoons caster/granulated sugar

4½ teaspoons gluten-free baking powder

a pinch of fine sea salt

¼ teaspoon xanthan gum

40 g/3 tablespoons salted butter, softened

140 ml/½ cup plus 1½ tablespoons buttermilk

1 egg

75 g/½ cup sultanas/golden raisins

1 beaten egg, to glaze

butter, jam/jelly and clotted cream, to serve

a straight-edged round cookie cutter (5–6 cm/2–2½ inches diameter)

1–2 baking sheets lined with baking parchment or silicone baking mats

makes 4–6

Preheat the oven to 190°C (375°F) Gas 5.

To a large bowl, or the bowl of a free-standing mixer, add the flour, sugar, baking powder, salt and xanthan gum. Add the softened butter to the dry ingredients in small pieces. Either rub in by hand or on a slow speed in a mixer until the mixture resembles breadcrumbs.

In a jug/pitcher, combine the buttermilk and egg, then pour into the dry mixture. Stir together using a large metal spoon or again on a slow speed if using a mixer. Once you have a sticky dough, stop mixing. At this point, quickly stir in the sultanas/golden raisins until evenly distributed.

Dust the work surface well with flour. Briefly knead the dough, then gently press into a flat disc 2–3-cm/1–1¼-inches thick. With the cookie cutter, stamp out scones from the dough. Push straight down and lift the cutter straight up, as twisting will prevent the scones from rising evenly. Briefly re-knead the remaining dough and stamp out more scones.

Space the scones on the prepared baking sheets to allow for spreading and rising. Brush the tops with the beaten egg to glaze, then bake in the preheated oven for 15–20 minutes until risen, golden and firm to the touch. Check the scones are done by carefully lifting and tapping the bottom – they should make a hollow sound. Cool the scones on a wire rack before serving – with butter, jam/jelly and clotted cream, of course!

Note
Scones are always best served as fresh as possible. If you are keeping them overnight, warm them for a few minutes in the oven before serving.

Variations
If you prefer your scones plain, simply omit the sultanas/golden raisins. Or swap in the same quantity of dried cranberries or chopped dried apricots, or the zest of 1 lemon and 1–2 tablespoons poppy seeds.

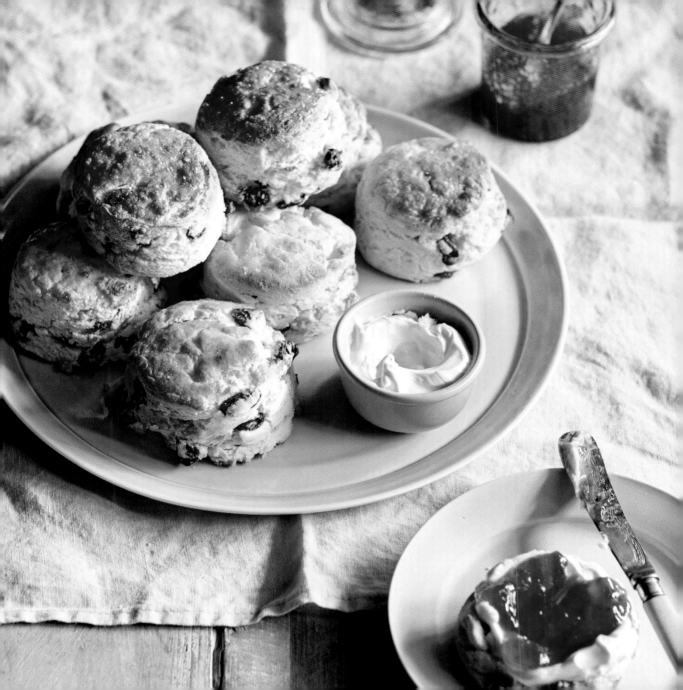

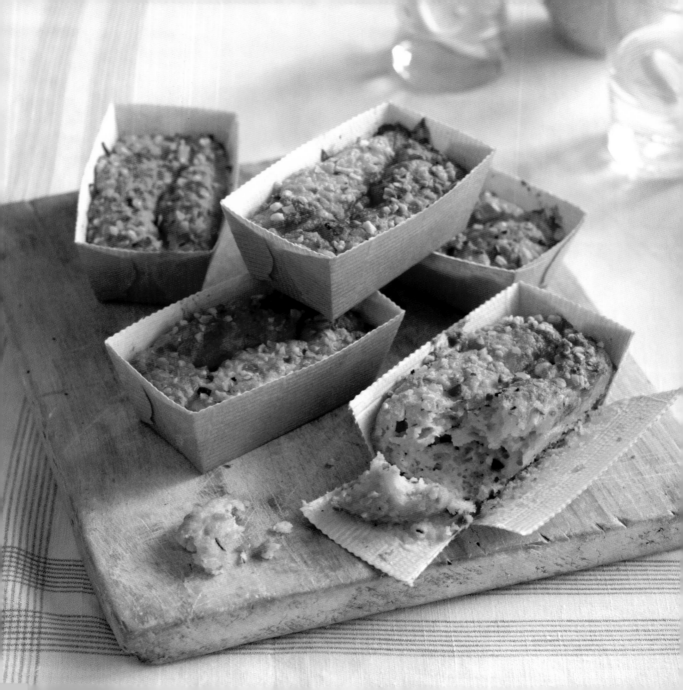

taleggio & hazelnut loaf cakes

115 g/1 stick butter, softened

1 tablespoon caster/granulated sugar

2 eggs

115 g self-raising/rising gluten-free flour OR scant 1 cup plain/all-purpose gluten-free flour plus 1 teaspoon gluten-free baking powder and ¾ teaspoon xanthan gum

200 g/7 oz. taleggio cheese, rind removed, chopped into small pieces

1 tablespoon crème fraîche or soured cream

1 courgette/zucchini, grated

2 tablespoons roasted and chopped hazelnuts

sea salt and freshly ground black pepper

8 mini loaf cases

makes 8

These loaf cakes are tangy from the creamy taleggio cheese, moist from the grated courgette/zucchini and have a great crunchy hazelnut topping. Delicious!

Preheat the oven to 180°C (350°F) Gas 4.

In a large mixing bowl, whisk together the butter, sugar, eggs and flour (plus baking powder and xanthan gum, if using). Add the taleggio pieces, crème fraîche (or soured cream) and grated courgette/zucchini to the mixture, season well with salt and pepper, and fold everything together.

Spoon the batter into the loaf cases, dividing evenly, and sprinkle the tops with chopped hazelnuts. Bake in the preheated oven for 25–30 minutes until the cakes are golden brown and spring back to your touch. Leave to cool before serving.

The cakes will keep for up to 2 days in an airtight container.

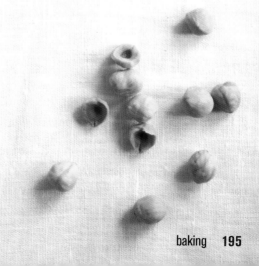

cheese & rosemary scones

These make an excellent lunch, served warm from the oven. They are also a novel accompaniment to a bowl of hot tomato soup; cold, they can be packed up for picnics. Any hard cheese can be grated or crumbled into the mix, and the herbs and spices varied to complement it. Try stilton and chive, manchego and basil or add 1 tablespoon of caster/granulated sugar instead of the mustard powder and give Wensleydale and dried cranberries a whirl.

225 g/1½ cups plain/all-purpose gluten-free flour, plus extra for dusting

4½ teaspoons gluten-free baking powder

½ teaspoon gluten-free mustard powder

¼ teaspoon sea salt

¼ teaspoon xanthan gum

40 g/3 tablespoons unsalted butter, softened

60 g/2 oz. (about ¾ cup) grated Cheddar cheese

2 tablespoons fresh rosemary leaves, finely chopped

140 ml/½ cup plus 1½ tablespoons buttermilk

1 egg

1 beaten egg, to glaze

butter and red onion marmalade, to serve (optional)

a straight-edged cookie cutter, 5–6 cm/2–2¼ inches in diameter

a baking sheet lined with baking parchment or a silicone baking mat

makes 4–6

Preheat the oven to 190°C (375°F) Gas 5.

To a large bowl, or the bowl of a free-standing mixer, add the flour, baking powder, mustard powder, salt and xanthan gum. Add the butter in small pieces. Either rub in by hand or on a slow speed in a mixer until the mixture resembles breadcrumbs and no large lumps of butter remain. Stir in the grated cheese and half the rosemary.

In a jug/pitcher, combine the buttermilk and whole egg, then pour into the dry mixture. Stir together using a large metal spoon or on a slow speed if using a mixer. Once you have a sticky dough, stop mixing.

Dust the work surface well with flour. Briefly knead the dough, then gently press into a flat disc 2–3-cm/1–1½-inches thick. Stamp out scones from the dough using the cookie cutter. Push straight down and lift the cutter straight up, as twisting will prevent the scones from rising evenly. Briefly re-knead the remaining dough and stamp out more scones.

Space the scones on the prepared baking sheet to allow for spreading and rising. Brush over the tops of the scones with the beaten egg to glaze, then sprinkle with the rest of the chopped rosemary.

Bake in the preheated oven for 15–20 minutes until risen, golden and firm to the touch. Gently lift a scone up from the sheet: the bottom should also be lightly browned and sound hollow when tapped. If required, return to the oven for 3–5 minutes more. Allow to cool slightly on a wire rack before serving with lashings of butter and perhaps some red onion marmalade. These scones are best eaten on the day they are made.

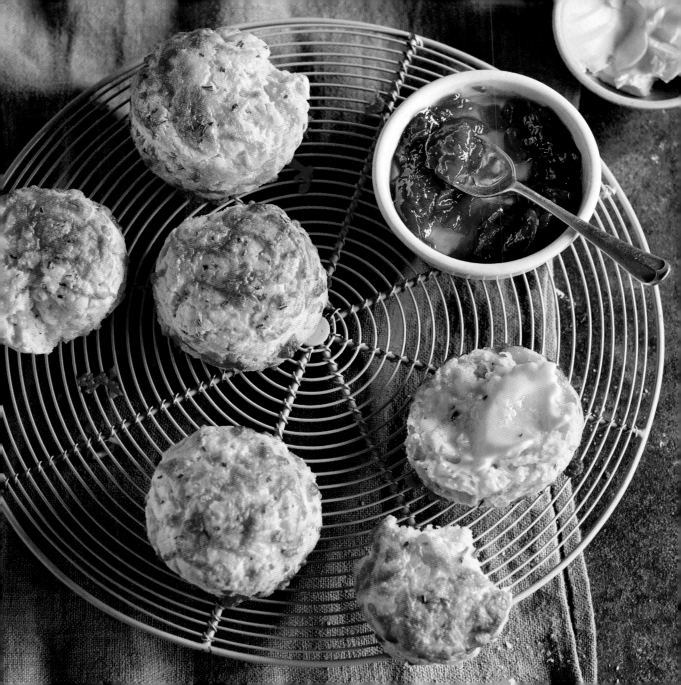

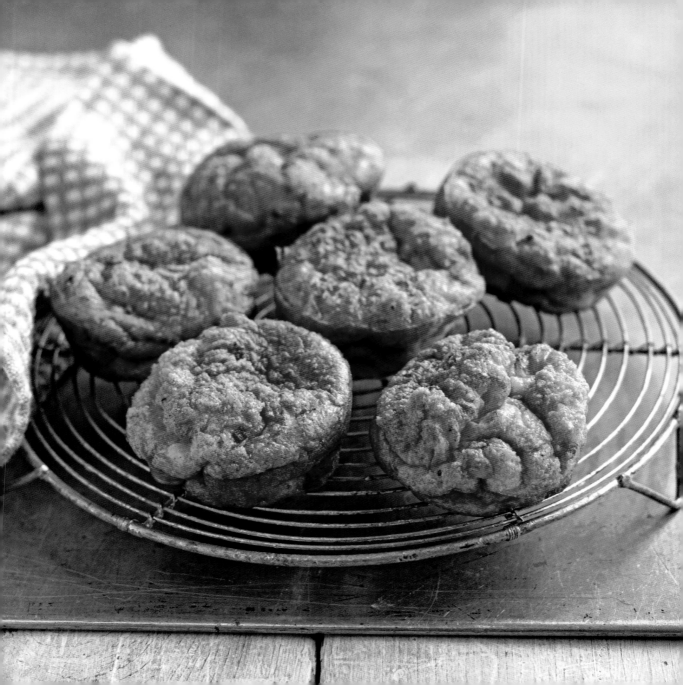

These muffins are quick and simple to prepare and are deliciously light and tasty. Needing only a few ingredients, they are a great standby recipe. To make them dairy-free as well, omit the cheese and replace with some corn kernels instead.

cheese & onion soufflé muffins

1 onion, finely chopped

1 tablespoon oil

5 eggs, separated

125 g/1¼ cups grated red Leicester or mature/sharp Cheddar cheese

sea salt and freshly ground black pepper

a 12-hole muffin pan, well-greased

makes 12

Preheat the oven to 180°C (350°F) Gas 4.

In a frying pan, cook the onion in the oil until softened and lightly golden brown, then leave to cool.

In a mixing bowl, stir together the egg yolks, cooked onion and grated cheese, and season with salt and pepper.

Put the egg whites in a separate bowl and whisk them to stiff peaks.

Gently fold the egg whites into the cheese mixture with a spatula until the cheese and onions are evenly distributed through the egg. Spoon the mixture into the holes of the muffin pan and bake in the preheated oven for 20–25 minutes until the soufflés have risen and are golden brown. Remove the muffins from the pan while still warm. These muffins are best served straight away.

for the scones

100 g/3½ oz. gluten-free spicy chorizo sausage

350 g self-raising/rising gluten-free flour plus 2 teaspoons gluten-free baking powder OR 2¾ cups plain/all-purpose gluten-free flour plus 5 teaspoons gluten-free baking powder and 2 teaspoons xanthan gum, plus extra flour for dusting

100 g/⅔ cup ground almonds

115 g/1 stick butter

100 g/3½ oz. Manchego cheese, cut into small cubes

200–250 ml/¾–1 cup milk, plus extra to glaze

paprika, to sprinkle

caster/granulated sugar, to sprinkle

sea salt and freshly ground black pepper

for the paprika butter

115 g/1 stick butter, softened

1 teaspoon sea salt flakes

1 teaspoon hot smoked paprika

an 8-cm/3½-inch triangle pastry cutter

a baking sheet, greased and lined with non-stick baking paper

makes 10

The spicy oil from the chorizo imparts its flavour into these delicious scones as they bake. Serve warm spread with paprika butter. Such whipped butters are a treat and well worth the effort.

chorizo & Manchego scones

Preheat the oven to 180°C (350°F) Gas 4.

Cut the chorizo into small pieces and dry-fry in a frying pan/skillet until the chorizo releases its oil and the edges start to turn crispy. Leave to cool.

Sift the flour and baking powder (plus xanthan gum, if using) into a large mixing bowl, add the ground almonds and butter and rub in the butter with your fingertips until the mixture resembles fine breadcrumbs. Add the cubes of Manchego to the flour mixture, along with the chorizo and any oil from the frying pan and season with a little salt and pepper. Gradually add the milk and bring together into a soft dough, adding a little more milk if needed.

On a flour-dusted surface, roll out the dough to about 2.5 cm/1 inch thick and stamp out the scones using the pastry cutter, re-rolling the trimmings as necessary. (You should only re-roll the dough once as it will become crumbly with the extra flour and difficult to roll.) Lay the scones on the prepared baking sheet, spacing them well apart. Use a pastry brush to brush the tops with a little extra milk, sprinkle with a little paprika and sugar. Bake in the preheated oven for 20–25 minutes until the tops are golden and the scones sound hollow when you tap them.

Make the paprika butter just before serving as it will lose its whipped texture if refrigerated. Whip the butter in a stand mixer or with an electric hand-held whisk for a few minutes with the salt and paprika until it is light and creamy. Serve the scones warm with the whipped butter.

The scones do not keep well and so are best eaten on the day they are made, or can be frozen and reheated to serve.

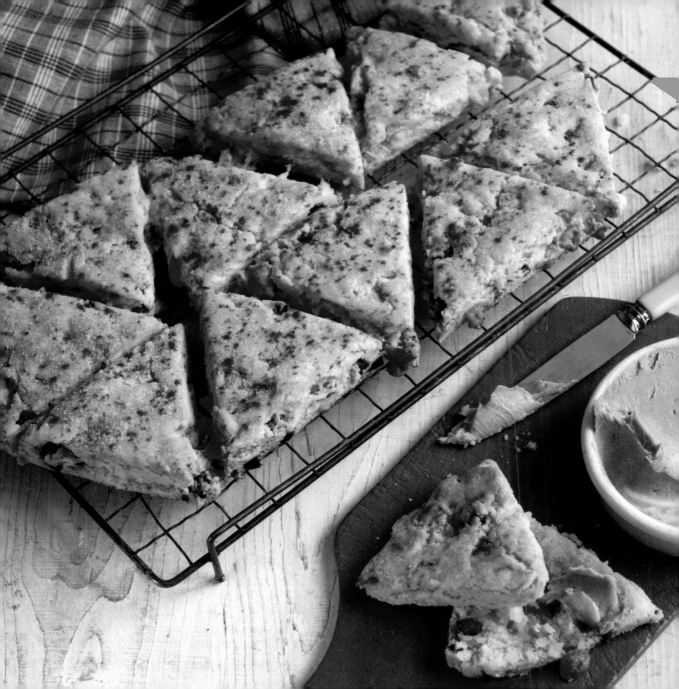

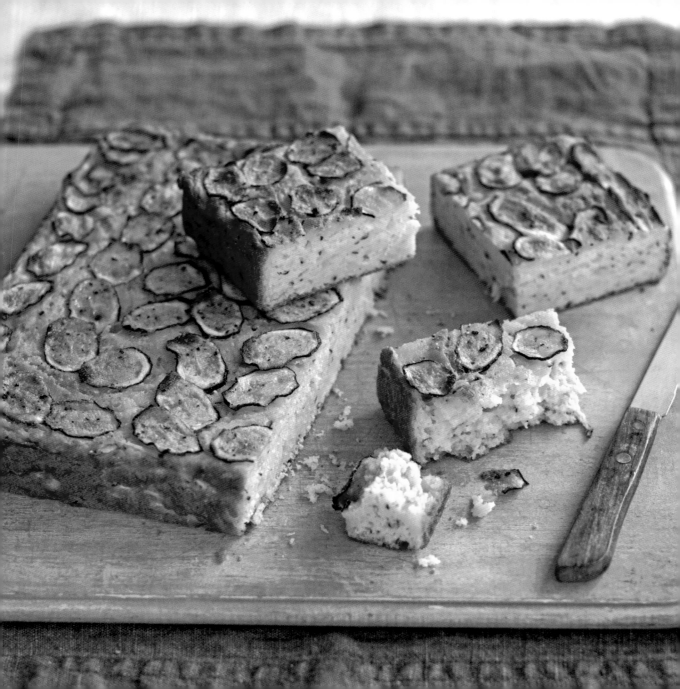

courgette bread

This tasty bread is perfect with soups and cheese. It has a pretty courgette/zucchini and a cornmeal topping, which gives the top of the loaf a nice crunchy coating. If you prefer blue cheese, you can substitute this for the Cheddar for a more piquant flavour.

200 g self-raising/rising gluten-free flour plus 3 teaspoons gluten-free baking powder OR 1²⁄₃ cups plain/all-purpose gluten-free flour plus 4¾ teaspoons gluten-free baking powder and 1¼ teaspoons xanthan gum

100 g/¾ cup fine cornmeal, plus extra for dusting

3 eggs, beaten

60 g/4 tablespoons butter, melted and cooled

300 ml/1¼ cups milk

150 g/5½ oz. Applewood smoked Cheddar, grated

2 courgettes/zucchini (about 350 g/12 oz.), ends trimmed

sea salt and freshly ground black pepper

olive oil, for brushing

a mandolin (optional)

a 24-cm/10-inch loose-based square cake pan, greased and lined with non-stick baking parchment

makes 1 loaf

Preheat the oven to 180°C (350°F) Gas 4.

Sift the flour, baking powder (plus xanthan gum, if using) and cornmeal into a large mixing bowl. Add the beaten eggs to the flour along with the melted butter and milk, then fold in the grated cheese.

Grate one of the courgettes/zucchini and add it to the mixture, folding everything together well. Season with salt and pepper, then spoon the mixture into the prepared cake pan.

Thinly slice the remaining courgette/zucchini using a mandoline or a sharp knife. Lay the courgette/zucchini slices in lines on top of the mixture in the pan and sprinkle over a little freshly ground black pepper. Dust the courgette/zucchini slices with cornmeal, then lightly dab the olive oil over the top of the loaf using a pastry brush.

Bake the bread in the preheated oven for 40–50 minutes, until the top is golden and the loaf springs back to your touch. Leave the loaf to cool in the pan for 5 minutes, then turn out onto a wire rack to cool completely.

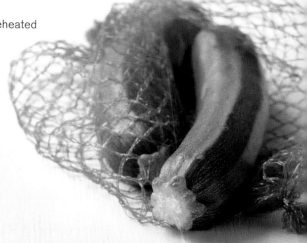

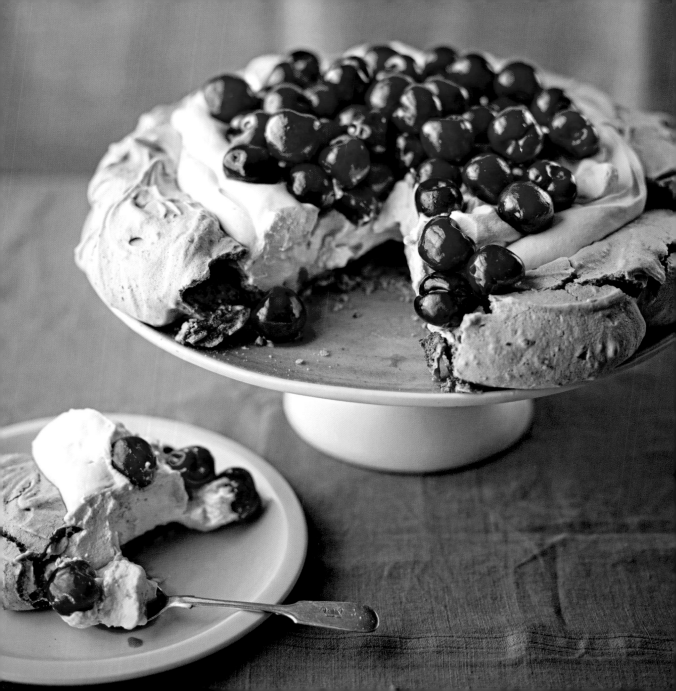

desserts

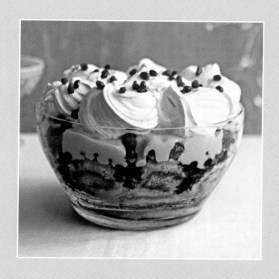

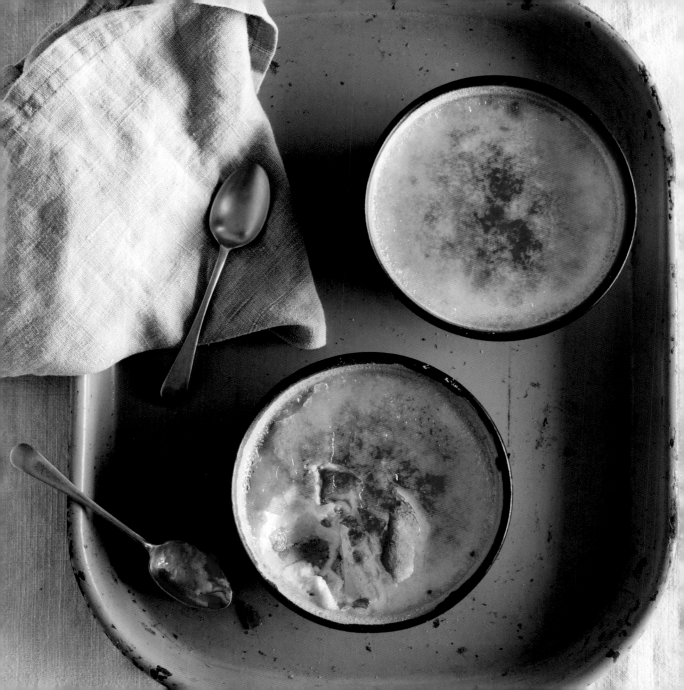

coconut crème brûlées

This is a gluten- and dairy-free version of a French classic, with a slightly tropical feel from the coconut cream. If you aren't avoiding dairy, the recipe works equally well with double/heavy cream.

25 g/2 tablespoons caster/granulated sugar, plus extra to sprinkle

3 egg yolks

1 vanilla pod/bean

300 ml/1 ¼ cups coconut cream

a chef's blowtorch (optional)

makes 2–3

Preheat the oven to 170°C (325°F) Gas 3.

Place 2 large, or 3 small, ramekins into a deep baking dish and set aside.

In a large jug/pitcher, whisk together the caster/granulated sugar and egg yolks. Remove the seeds from the vanilla pod/bean (by splitting open the pod/bean lengthways and carefully running the blade of a knife along the inside of each half), add to the mixture and whisk again.

Put the coconut cream in a pan set over a low heat until simmering. Pour the cream into the jug/pitcher with the eggs, whisking all the time, until well combined. Pour the mixture into the ramekins until nearly full.

Pour some tepid water into the baking dish containing the filled ramekins until it reaches halfway up the sides of the ramekins, then put the whole lot into the preheated oven to bake for 30–35 minutes.

Check that the brûlées are set by giving the dish a gentle shake. There should be just a slight wobble to the custards. Remove from the oven and allow to cool before putting into the fridge for a couple of hours to chill and set completely.

When you are ready to serve, sprinkle the tops of the brûlées with caster/granulated sugar. Ideally, use a chef's blowtorch to caramelize the sugar, swirling the ramekins around as you melt the sugar so that it creates an even layer of crunchy caramel. If you don't have a blowtorch, preheat the grill/broiler to hot and place the brûlées underneath. If the custards get too hot, you can pop them back into the fridge to re-chill before serving.

Note
Coconut cream can be found in larger supermarkets, but if you can't find it, buy two cans of regular coconut milk and allow them to settle in a cool place for a few hours. The coconut cream and coconut water will separate in the can. Open, and spoon off the cream, discarding the water beneath.

peach cobbler

8 large, ripe peaches

50 g/¼ cup caster/granulated sugar

1 tablespoon plain/all-purpose gluten-free flour

1 teaspoon freshly squeezed lemon juice

pouring cream, to serve

for the cobbler topping

260 g/1¾ cups plain/all-purpose gluten-free flour

60 g/¼ cup plus 1 tablespoon caster/granulated sugar

4 teaspoons gluten-free baking powder

½ teaspoon xanthan gum

a pinch of fine sea salt

150 ml/⅔ cup natural/plain yogurt

60 g/4 tablespoons unsalted butter, melted

2 eggs, beaten

a 20-cm/8-inch round baking pan

serves 4–6

Cobbler is a kind of stateside crumble. It's a fabulous summer dessert, and easy to whip up. Use really ripe peaches, or nectarines if you prefer, and serve with cream, custard or ice cream. You can vary the fruits if you like as well – an apricot or blackberry version are both utterly delicious.

Preheat the oven to 190°C (375°F) Gas 5.

Halve and stone/pit the peaches and thinly slice them. Toss in a bowl with the caster/granulated sugar, flour and lemon juice, then spread evenly over the base of the baking pan.

Bake in the preheated oven for 10–15 minutes.

For the cobbler topping, mix together the flour, sugar, baking powder, xanthan gum and a pinch of salt in a large bowl. Make a well in the centre of the mixture and pour in the yogurt, melted butter and three-quarters of the beaten eggs (reserve one quarter for glazing the top of the cobbler). Stir everything together until it comes together in a wet dough and set aside for a minute or so.

Remove the peaches from the oven, give the cobbler topping another stir and then dollop 6–8 large spoonfuls of the mixture onto the fruit, spacing evenly apart. The topping will spread as it bakes, so all of the fruit doesn't need to be covered.

Lightly brush the tops of the dough with the remaining beaten egg and return the dish to the oven to bake for 30–35 minutes until the cobbler is golden and feels firm when gently pressed.

Remove from the oven and allow to cool for a few minutes before serving with pouring cream.

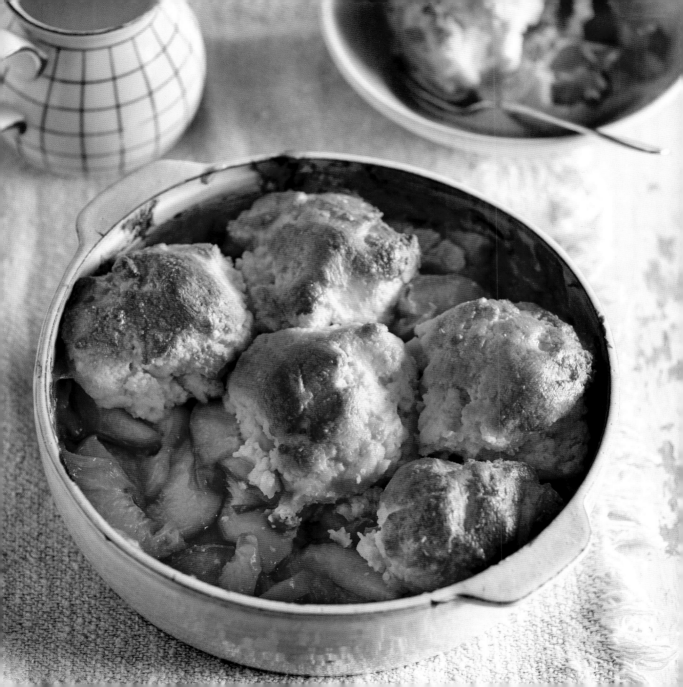

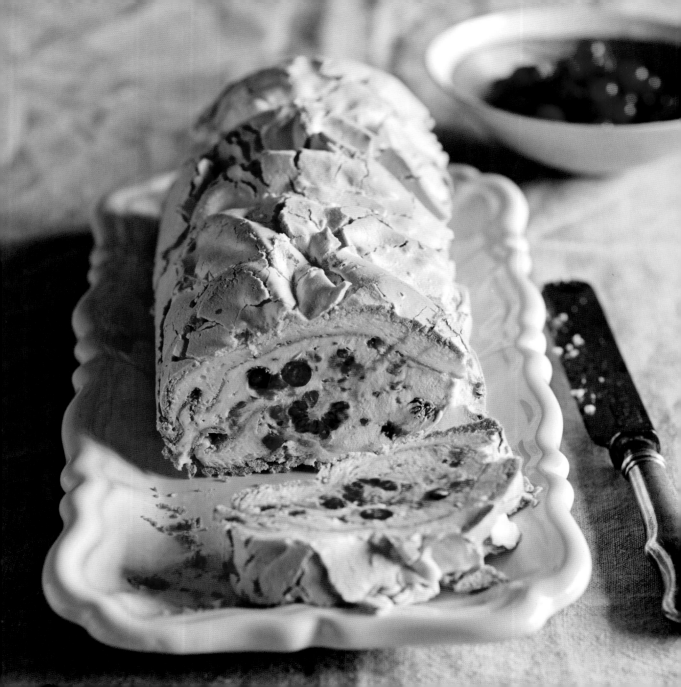

Making a roulade can challenge any baker. A good dusting of icing/confectioners' sugar should fix the inevitable cracking.

raspberry & redcurrant roulade

5 egg whites

275 g/1⅓ cups caster/superfine sugar

1 teaspoon white wine vinegar

1 teaspoon cornflour/cornstarch

2 tablespoons gluten-free icing/confectioners' sugar, plus extra for dusting

300 ml/1¼ cups double/heavy cream

200 g/1⅓ cups fresh raspberries

150 g/1 cup fresh redcurrants

a Swiss/jelly roll pan lined with baking parchment

serves 8–12

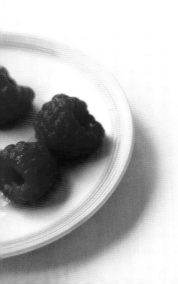

Preheat the oven to 200°C (400°F) Gas 6.

In a spotlessly clean bowl, whisk the egg whites until they are stiff. Add the sugar, a heaped tablespoon at a time, whisking until fully incorporated. Once all the sugar has been added, the meringue should be very thick and shiny. Whisk in the white wine vinegar and cornflour/cornstarch.

Using a spatula, spoon the mixture onto the baking parchment in the Swiss/jelly roll pan and spread out evenly. Bake in the preheated oven for 10 minutes, then, without opening the door, turn the heat down to 170°C (325°F) Gas 3 and bake for a further 15–20 minutes until crisp and firm. Remove the pan from the oven and leave to cool for 10 minutes.

Take a chopping board larger than your pan and lay onto it a clean kitchen cloth followed by a fresh piece of baking parchment. Dust the top of the meringue in the pan with icing/confectioners' sugar and then place the board over the pan so that the parchment meets the meringue. Invert the whole thing, then place onto a work surface and carefully lift away the pan. Allow to cool completely.

When the meringue has cooled, whisk the double/heavy cream and the 2 tablespoons of icing/confectioners' sugar until quite thick, then fold in most of the raspberries. Strip half of the redcurrant berries from their stalks and fold these in as well. Remove the parchment from the underside of the meringue and spread the cream and berry mixture evenly over the top.

Use the kitchen cloth and baking parchment to roll the meringue into a log shape – try to do so quite tightly, and don't worry if it cracks a little. Transfer to a serving plate or board and chill in the fridge before serving. To serve, garnish the top of the roulade with the remaining raspberries and redcurrants and dust generously with icing/confectioners' sugar.

This has to be one of the simplest desserts to make, and as such it's perfect for days when you are pushed for time. You can make them look extra special by serving them in some pretty glasses or vintage china tea cups, but small ramekins are fine too. Garnish them with some candied lemon zest.

lemon possets

3 large lemons
400 ml/1¾ cups double/heavy cream
125 g/⅔ cup caster/granulated sugar

for the candied peel
1 lemon
70 g/⅓ cup caster/granulated sugar

makes 4

Finely zest 1 lemon and put the zest into a saucepan along with the cream and sugar.

Juice all of the lemons (including the one that has been zested) and set to one side, ensuring that there are no pips in the juice.

Over a low heat, bring the cream, sugar and lemon zest to a simmer for 2 minutes. Remove from the heat and whisk in the lemon juice.

Divide the mixture evenly between four glasses, tea cups or ramekins. Put in the fridge and allow to set for a minimum of 3 hours before serving.

While the possets set, make the candied peel for decoration.

Peel the lemon rind in long strips and use a sharp knife to remove any white pith from the underside. Slice into thin strips and put into a saucepan with the sugar and 200 ml/¾ cup of water. Heat the mixture over a low heat, stirring just until the sugar is dissolved, and then bring to a simmer. Simmer for 15–20 minutes until the strips of zest are almost translucent and the liquid has reduced by at least two-thirds.

Remove the pan from the heat and use a fork to lift the zest strips from the pan. Spread onto a baking sheet or plate in a single layer and leave uncovered to cool and set.

When you are ready to serve, take a few strips of candied peel and arrange on top of the now-set lemon possets.

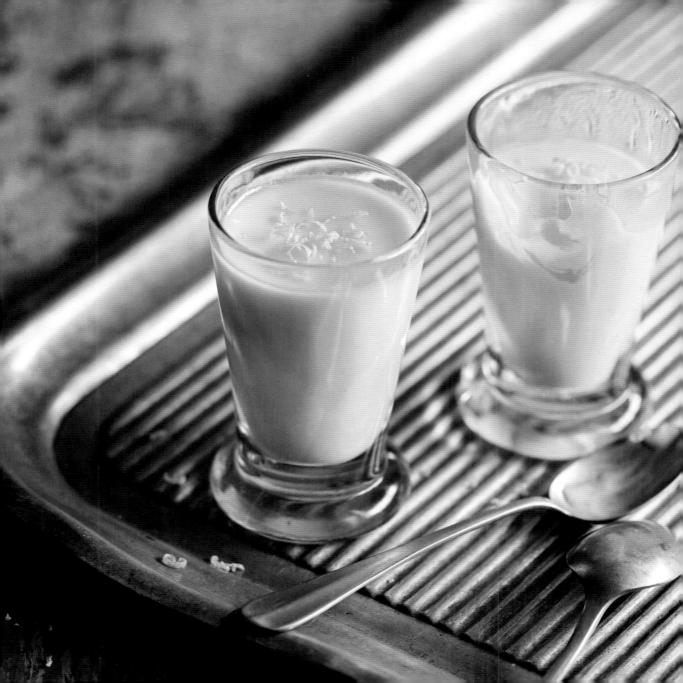

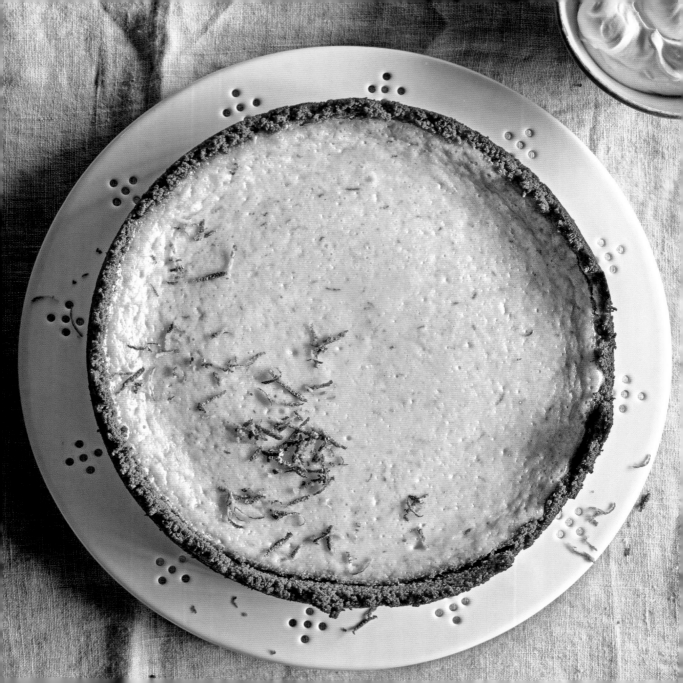

key lime pie

Although this recipe takes its name from the Florida Keys' limes that it is traditionally made with, any fresh, juicy limes will do just fine. Zingy and light, it makes a wonderful dinner-party dessert, as it can be made ahead and stored in the fridge until serving.

175 g/1½ sticks unsalted butter, melted

300 g/10½ oz. gluten-free digestive biscuits/graham crackers (see Note)

3 egg yolks

grated zest and freshly squeezed juice of 4 large limes

1 x 397-g/14-oz. can sweetened condensed milk

350 ml/scant 1½ cups double/heavy cream

2 tablespoons gluten-free icing/confectioners' sugar

a 23-cm/9-inch springform tart pan lightly greased with melted butter

serves 8

Preheat the oven to 180°C (350°F) Gas 4.

To begin, make the base. This is most easily done using a food processor: put the biscuits/graham crackers into it and whizz until they are in fine crumbs. Pour in the melted butter and mix until completely combined. You can make the base by hand by placing the biscuits in a plastic food bag wrapped in a kitchen towel and bashing with a rolling pin until you reach a crumb consistency, then transfer to a mixing bowl and stir in the melted butter with a wooden spoon. Press the mixture evenly into the bottom and halfway up the sides of the prepared tart pan. Bake in the preheated oven for 10 minutes, then remove and set aside to cool. Keep the oven on.

To a large bowl, or the bowl of a free-standing mixer, add the egg yolks and lime zest, reserving a little to garnish if desired. Whisk together for a minute and then add the lime juice and condensed milk. Whisk for 3–4 minutes until smooth. Pour the topping onto the now slightly cooled biscuit/graham cracker base, then put the whole thing back into the oven and bake for 15–20 minutes until the mixture feels set. Remove from the oven, put the pan onto a wire rack and allow to cool for at least an hour. Refrigerate for a further 3 hours, minimum, but preferably overnight.

When ready to serve, gently remove the pie from the pan and transfer to a serving plate. Whip the double/heavy cream with the icing/confectioners' sugar until standing in soft peaks. Serve the cream separately or dress the pie with clouds of whipped or piped cream. Add some lime zest, if you like.

Note
If you can't find digestives, any plain gluten-free biscuit will work here. If you are using an unsweetened cracker style biscuit, add a few tablespoons of caster/granulated sugar before the melted butter.

8 medium dessert apples

40 g/3 tablespoons caster/granulated sugar

1 tablespoon plain/all-purpose gluten-free flour

1 teaspoon ground cinnamon

pouring cream or dairy-free ice cream, to serve

for the crumble topping

70 g/5 tablespoons unsalted butter or dairy-free spread, softened

140 g/1 scant cup plain/all-purpose gluten-free flour

a pinch of fine sea salt

70 g/⅓ cup caster/granulated sugar

1 teaspoon ground cinnamon

a 20-cm/8-inch baking dish

serves 4–6

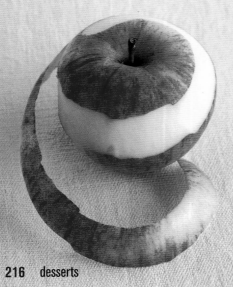

apple crumble

A crumble warrants little by way of introduction. Once you've cracked this recipe – and it really is gloriously simple – why not mix it up with different fruits and spices – pear and ginger, apple and blackberry, rhubarb and vanilla? You can be a bit cheffy about things, too! Mix up the crumble topping separately beforehand and bake on a lined baking sheet. Once cooled, blitz in a food processor. When ready to serve, take any warm, stewed fruit, pop it into a bowl and generously sprinkle over the crumble topping. Pop the dish under the hot grill/broiler for a few minutes and you'll have an almost instant crumble.

Preheat the oven to 190°C (375°F) Gas 5.

Peel and core the apples, then chop into 2-cm/¾-inch chunks. Toss the apples with a tablespoon of water, the caster/granulated sugar, flour and cinnamon, then spread evenly over the base of the baking dish. Press down lightly with your hands.

To make the crumble topping, rub together the butter (or dairy-free spread) and flour and a pinch of salt until the mixture resembles rough breadcrumbs. Stir in the sugar and cinnamon, then spread the mixture over the apples in the dish. Lightly press down the mixture so it is compact. (You can make the topping using a food processor, if you have one. Put all of the ingredients in at the same time and pulse until you have a consistency similar to breadcrumbs.)

Put the dish onto a baking sheet and bake in the preheated oven for 40–45 minutes until the crumble is golden and just browning on top. Remove from the oven and allow to cool for a few minutes before serving with pouring cream or dairy-free ice cream.

Note
To make this crumble dairy-free as well, simply substitute the butter in the crumble topping for your preferred dairy-free spread and serve with dairy-free ice cream.

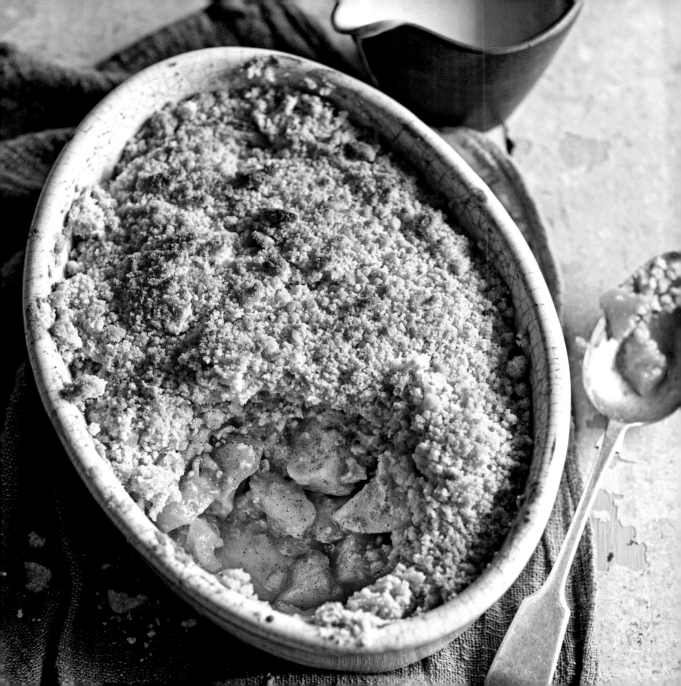

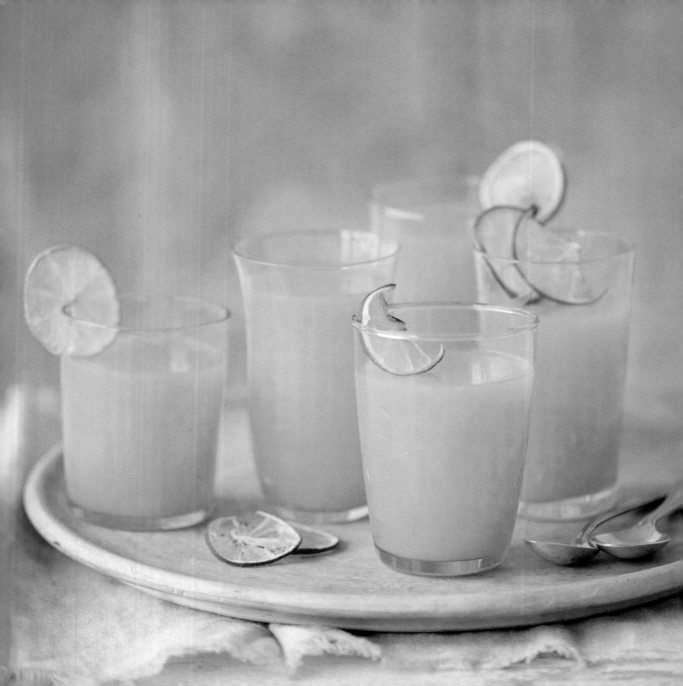

2 large ripe mangoes, stoned/pitted, peeled and roughly chopped

7 tablespoons caster/granulated sugar

20 g leaf gelatine/4 x gelatin sheets

5 tablespoons Muscat dessert wine

3 tablespoons freshly squeezed lime juice

finely grated zest of 1 lime

to serve

zest of 1 lime, or thin lime slices dried in a low oven

200 ml/scant 1 cup single/light cream (optional)

makes 4

Colourful, light and delicious, a classic combination after a large meal. Serve with lime relish and cream if desired.

mango & lime jellies

Purée the mango flesh in a food processor with the sugar until smooth.

Place the purée in a medium saucepan and heat gently.

Soak the gelatine in plenty of cold water for 5 minutes. Drain and squeeze the gelatine and place in the pan with the mango purée. Stir until dissolved. Add 500 ml/2 cups water, the dessert wine, lime juice and zest.

Mix thoroughly, pour into four tall glasses and chill for approximately 6 hours until set.

Serve decorated with extra lime zest (or dried lime slices) and cream, if desired.

An elderflower fizz jelly makes a delightfully light end to a meal and looks particularly elegant when adorned with fresh redcurrants. Add a sprinkle of popping candy just before serving for extra fizz. If you prefer not to include alcohol, substitute sparkling white grape juice or lemonade.

elderflower fizz jelly

250 ml/1 cup Prosecco

2 sheets large-leaf gelatine (if using small-leaf gelatine, use 4 pieces)

100 ml/6 tablespoons elderflower cordial

100 g/⅔ cup fresh raspberries

for the decorations (optional)

bunches of redcurrants

popping candy

makes 3–4

Pour the Prosecco into a jug/pitcher and get the serving glasses ready – either flutes, tumblers or small wine glasses, or even lightly oiled dariole moulds so you can turn the jellies out onto a plate before serving.

Fill a large bowl with water and fully submerge the gelatine sheets. Set aside to soften.

Put the elderflower cordial and 50 ml/3 tablespoons of water into a small saucepan and bring to a simmer over a medium heat. Remove the pan from the heat. Lift the gelatine sheets out of the water, give them a squeeze and then drop into the hot elderflower liquid. Stir until melted.

Pour the elderflower mixture into the jug/pitcher with the Prosecco and stir well. Set aside for a couple of minutes to cool slightly.

Place a few raspberries into each glass, stir the jelly mix again and pour into the glasses over the berries. Push any fruit that pops up over the jelly back into the liquid so everything is fully submerged and put the glasses into the fridge to set for 2–3 hours. (During the first 30 minutes, keep checking the fruit and prod it down into the jelly so that the berries are suspended in the mixture when set.)

For added pizzazz, you can drape a bunch of redcurrants over the top of each glass and sprinkle a little popping candy onto the surface of each jelly.

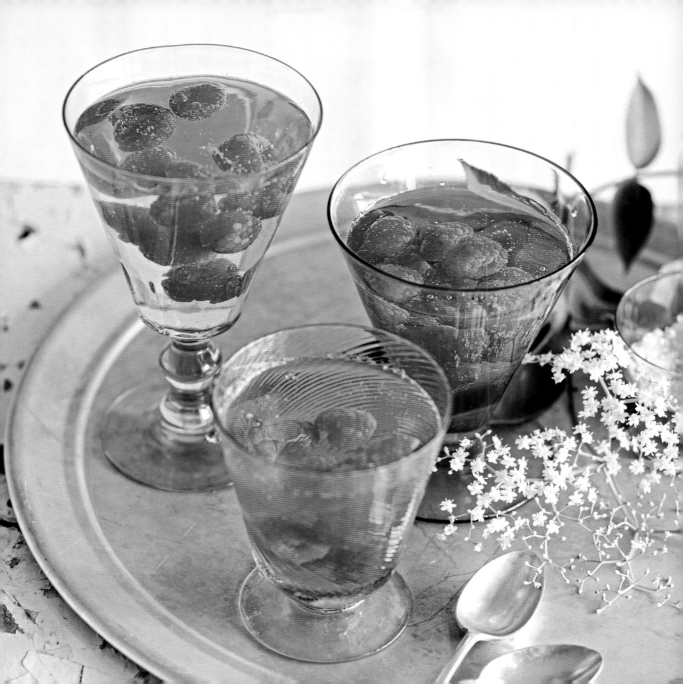

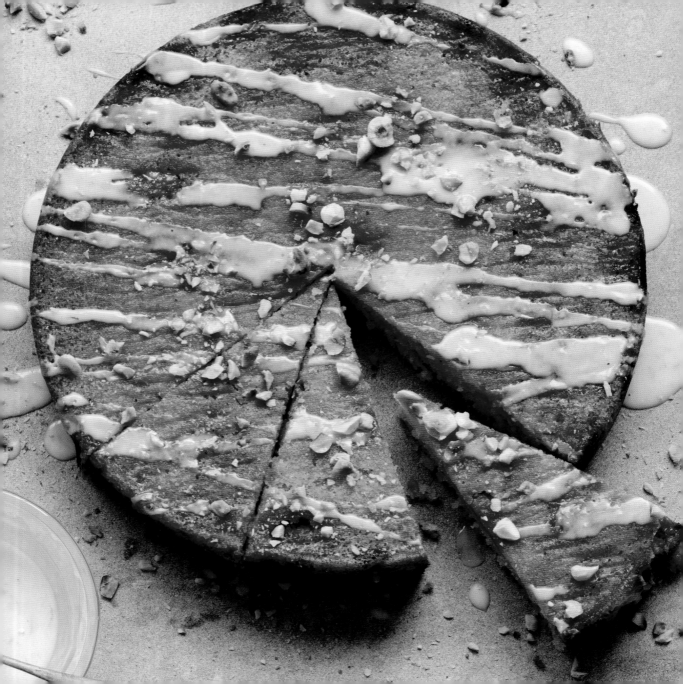

125 g/1 ⅛ sticks unsalted butter, softened

200 g/1 cup golden caster/granulated sugar

10 cardamom pods, seeds crushed

finely grated zest of 1 lemon

2 teaspoons vanilla extract

3 large eggs

200 g/1 cup fresh raspberries or blueberries

250 g/1 ½ cups ground almonds

a pinch of fine sea salt

1 teaspoon gluten-free baking powder

for the lemon drizzle icing

grated zest and freshly squeezed juice of 1 small lemon

200 g/1 ½ cups gluten-free icing/confectioners' sugar

handful of toasted hazelnuts, finely chopped

a 23-cm/9-inch springform cake pan, greased and lined with baking parchment

serves 6–8

lemon cardamom & raspberry torte

This recipe offers further proof that flourless cakes can be divine. Blueberries work as well as raspberries here. Why not serve this torte at the end of a dinner party with dessert wine?

Preheat the oven to 170°C (325°F) Gas 3.

Cream together the butter, sugar, cardamom seeds, lemon zest and vanilla extract until pale and fluffy. Add the eggs one at a time and beat between each addition.

Fold in the fruit, ground almonds, salt and baking powder. When everything is mixed together, fill the prepared cake pan with the mixture and bake in the preheated oven for 45 minutes until golden, and a skewer inserted into the centre comes out cleanly. Cool on a wire rack and then unmould.

To make the lemon drizzle icing, in a bowl, mix the lemon zest and juice with the icing/confectioners' sugar. Drizzle over the cooled torte and sprinkle with toasted hazelnuts, then cut and serve.

chocolate & pistachio cake with salted caramel

250 g/9 oz. dark/bittersweet chocolate, minimum 70% cocoa solids

225 g/1 cup sunflower butter

100 g/⅔ cup shelled unsalted pistachio nuts, plus 3 tablespoons, to serve

100 g/⅔ cup stoned/pitted Medjool dates

6 eggs

300 g/1½ cups coconut palm sugar

sea salt

1 teaspoon pure vanilla extract

200 ml/¾ cup coconut milk

unsweetened cocoa powder, to dust

a 23-cm/9 inch-loose-bottomed cake pan, greased and lined with baking parchment

serves 12

Surely the phrase 'death by chocolate' must have been dreamt up by someone eating a cake like this? It is so rich and decadent that there is every possibility you might just keel over upon tasting it, completely overcome by the chocolatey goodness.

Preheat the oven to 160°C (325°F), Gas 4.

Melt the chocolate and sunflower butter in a heatproof bowl over barely simmering water. While that is melting, place the pistachio nuts in a food processor and blitz until very finely ground. Remove to a bowl. Add the Medjool dates and two of the eggs to the processor and blitz until the dates are finely chopped. Remove to a separate bowl and whisk in the remaining four eggs. Set aside.

When the chocolate and butter have completely melted, whisk in 200 g/1 cup of the coconut palm sugar and ¼ teaspoon of salt while still sitting over the simmering water. Once dissolved, remove from the heat and whisk in the vanilla extract and the egg and date mixture. Make sure to whisk very quickly and continuously until the eggs have fully incorporated, resulting in a thick, shiny mixture, otherwise the eggs will be lumpy. Add the ground pistachio nuts and mix well to combine.

Pour into the prepared cake pan and bake in the centre of the oven for about 35 minutes or until the cake is set but with a little wobble in the centre. Leave to cool completely, then remove from the pan.

For the caramel, place a saucepan with the coconut milk and remaining 100 g/½ cup coconut palm sugar over a medium-high heat. Bring to the boil, stirring all the time, then reduce the heat, add in a large pinch of sea salt and simmer for 10 minutes, stirring on and off, until you have a thick and viscous caramel. Roughly chop the remaining pistachio nuts.

To serve, dust the cake with cocoa powder, pour over the caramel and sprinkle with the pistachio nuts and a little sea salt. Serve in thin slices.

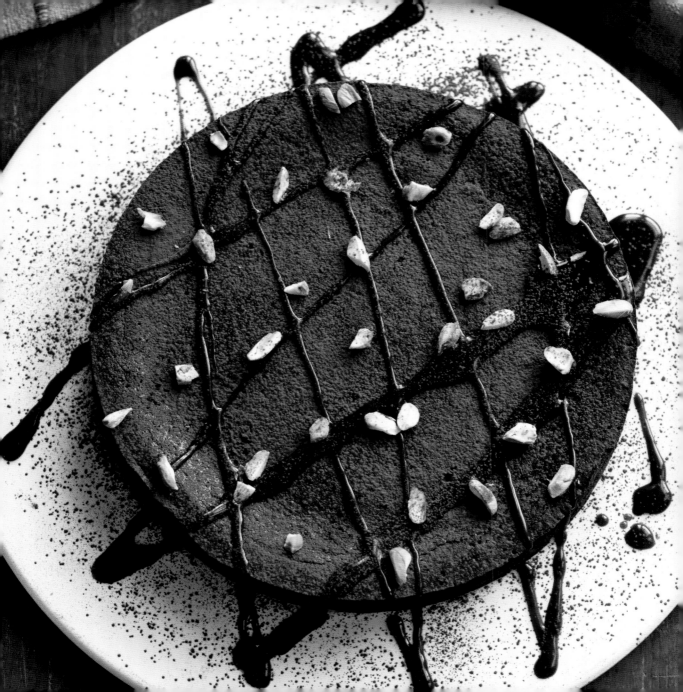

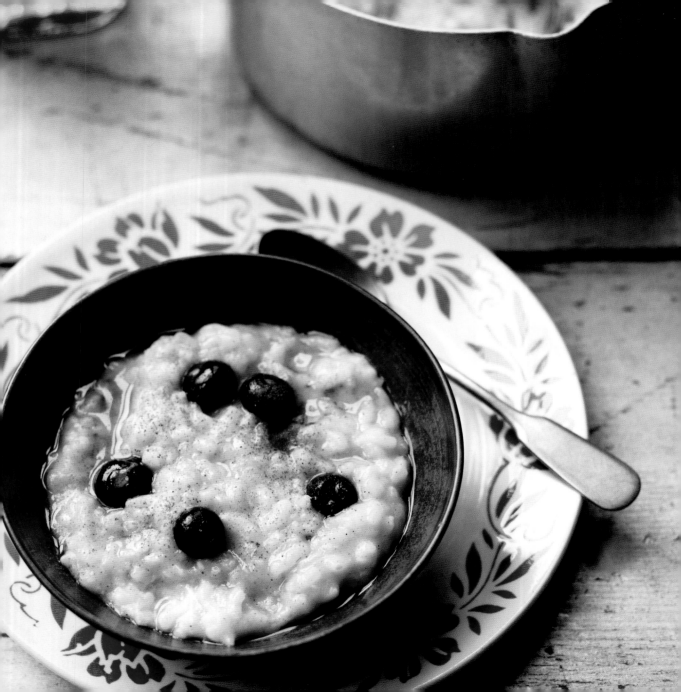

This luscious and thick dairy-free rice pudding is made using coconut milk and cream, and rice milk. For the toppings, feel free to use whatever you like. Medjool dates and nut butter swirled through the pudding work well.

coconut rice pudding with blueberries & maple syrup

150 g/¾ cup risotto rice, such as carnaroli or arborio

400-ml/14-fl. oz. can coconut milk

600 ml/2½ cups rice or almond milk

1 teaspoon vanilla extract

½ teaspoon ground cinnamon

a good pinch of freshly grated nutmeg, about ¼ teaspoon

a pinch of sea salt

3 tablespoons pure maple syrup, plus extra for drizzling

handful of frozen blueberries

serves 4

Rinse the rice thoroughly under cold running water and add to a pot with the coconut milk and rice or almond milk and bring to the boil. Reduce the heat to low and simmer gently for about 20–35 minutes, stirring regularly to ensure the rice does not stick to the bottom. By this stage the rice should be cooked through with a thick and creamy consistency. Stir in the vanilla extract, cinnamon, nutmeg, salt and maple syrup and taste, adding a little more of anything you particularly like.

When you are ready to serve, ladle the hot rice into bowls and add in a few frozen blueberries (or whatever topping you choose), straight from the freezer. Drizzle over a little extra maple syrup and serve immediately. The blueberries will thaw in the hot pudding, leaving gorgeous inky pools of juice.

300 g/10½ oz. dark/bittersweet chocolate

160 ml/⅔ cup coconut cream (the solidified coconut from a can of coconut milk or cream, see Note, page 207)

2 egg yolks

2 tablespoons palm sugar

2 tablespoons very strong coffee (or coffee extract), cooled

1–2 tablespoons rum (optional)

3 egg whites

chopped hazelnuts, toasted to garnish

cacao (or cocoa) nibs, to garnish

serves 4

This mousse works well served in coffee cups, and topped with chopped hazelnuts and ground cacao beans. You can exchange the coffee and rum (if using) with things like citrus juice and grated zest, or raspberries if you fancy a change.

mocha mousse

Break the chocolate up into a heatproof bowl. Warm the coconut cream in a saucepan over a medium heat and pour over the chocolate to melt. Leave for 5 minutes, stirring occasionally. If the chocolate hasn't completely melted, set the bowl over a pan of simmering water for a moment or two. You want to heat the chocolate as little as possible.

In a separate bowl, whisk together the egg yolks and the palm sugar until light and creamy.

Once the chocolate is cool, but still melted, add this to the egg yolk and sugar mixture with the coffee and rum (if using) and stir until well combined.

In a third bowl, whisk the egg whites using a hand-held electric whisk until you have soft peaks. Use a slotted spoon to fold the egg whites into the chocolate mixture.

Spoon the mixture into coffee cups, serving dishes or one large dish. Put in the fridge to set for 2–3 hours.

Top with chopped toasted hazelnuts and cacao nibs to decorate, and to serve.

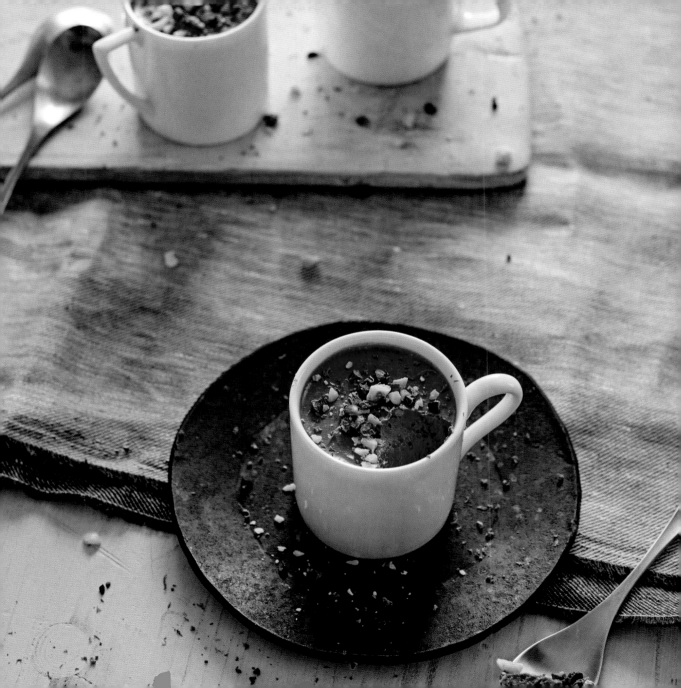

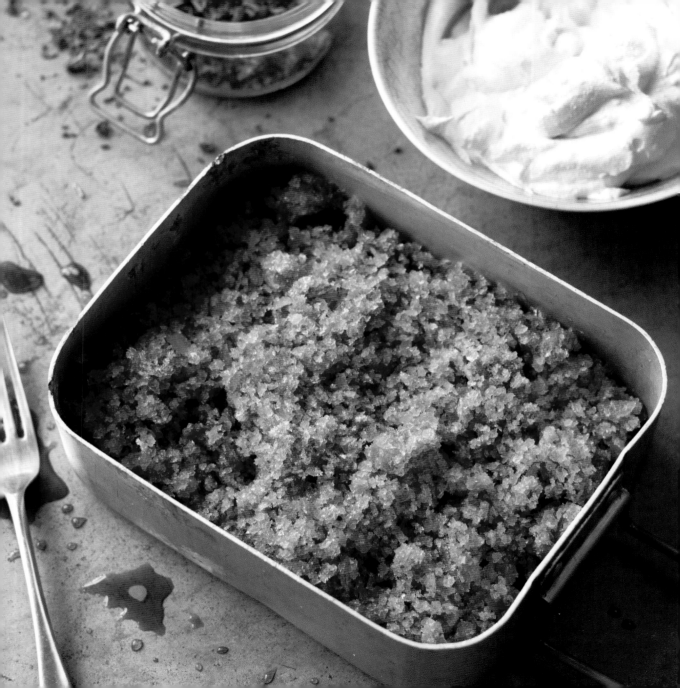

coffee granita with whipped coconut cream

for the granita

250 ml/1 cup water

45 g/¼ cup demerara/turbinado sugar

3 tablespoons coffee substitute (Yannoh, Bianca or Orzo), plus extra to serve

1 tablespoon coffee extract

¼ teaspoon bourbon vanilla powder

for the whipped coconut cream

150 ml/generous ½ cup coconut cream (see Note on page 207 if you can't find coconut cream)

1 tablespoon demerara/turbinado sugar

shaved dark/bittersweet chocolate, to serve

serves 3–4

If you are not a coffee drinker, but like the taste of coffee in cakes and desserts, you'll find that coffee substitutes are similar in taste, but without the side effects, so this dessert can be served to kids as well. The taste of coconut takes this dessert to another level of yumminess.

To make the granita, mix the water and sugar in a saucepan and bring to the boil. Whisk in the coffee substitute and let boil again. Remove from heat and add the coffee extract and vanilla. Leave to cool completely, pour into a shallow dish and put in the freezer for 15 minutes.

Whisk with a fork to distribute the frozen parts and break up the crystals. Freeze again until icy at the edge of pan and the overall texture is slushy, about 25 minutes. Whisk with a fork, put back in the freezer and whisk again after 20 minutes to distribute the frozen portions evenly. Cover and return to the freezer. When ready to serve, remove from the freezer and scrape the granita with a fork, forming icy flakes. You can make granita a couple of days ahead.

To make the whipped coconut cream, place the coconut cream in a tall and narrow bowl. With a freestanding mixer (or an electric hand-held whisk), whip on high speed for 2–3 minutes until it starts getting thicker. Add the sugar and whip for another 3–5 minutes. Be patient! Sometimes the cream gets soft peaks, and sometimes it stays fluffy. In any case, it is very tasty! If you want the cream to be snow-white, use icing/confectioners' sugar instead of demerara/turbinado sugar.

To serve, scoop the granita into parfait glasses, top with the whipped coconut cream and sprinkle with coffee substitute or shaved chocolate, as preferred. Serve immediately.

black forest pavlova

6 egg whites

a pinch of fine sea salt

335 g/1⅔ cups caster/superfine sugar

20 g/2½ tablespoons cocoa powder, sifted

1 teaspoon white wine vinegar

75 g/3½ oz. dark/bittersweet chocolate (60–70% cocoa solids), grated

600 ml/2½ cups double/heavy cream

for the kirsch-soaked cherries

600 g/4 cups stoned/pitted fresh cherries

3 tablespoons caster/granulated sugar

5–6 tablespoons kirsch (or other cherry liqueur)

a large baking sheet lined with baking parchment

serves 8

Pavlova was created in the 1920s in honour of the ballet dancer Anna Pavlova. Since no-one can agree whether it is an Australian or New Zealand invention, we've added Germany into the equation, giving it the Black Forest treatment.

Preheat the oven to 150°C (300°F) Gas 2.

Whisk the egg whites with the salt until stiff peaks form. Gradually, 1 tablespoon at a time, add the sugar, whisking between each addition. The meringue should be very stiff and glossy. Whisk in the cocoa and vinegar and fold in the chocolate with a large metal spoon.

Spoon generous dollops of meringue in a ring shape about 25 cm/10 in. in diameter onto the prepared baking sheet. Spoon more of the mixture in the middle and build up the sides slightly higher. Make swirls in the meringue using a fork for an attractive finish. Pop the meringue in the preheated oven, close the oven door and immediately reduce the temperature to 140°C (275°F) Gas 1. Bake for 1 hour.

Turn the oven off, but leave the meringue inside, with the oven door shut, until the oven is completely cold. It's easiest to make the meringue in the evening and leave it in the oven overnight to cool.

For the kirsch-soaked cherries, put the cherries in a bowl and sprinkle the sugar over the top. Pour in the kirsch and toss until all the cherries are completely coated. Cover the bowl with clingfilm/plastic wrap and leave to macerate for a few hours or even overnight while the meringue is also cooling.

Whip the cream in a bowl until stiff but not dry and whisk in 3–4 tablespoons of the macerating liquor from the cherries. Place the meringue on a cake stand and spread the cream thickly over the top, before piling on the drained cherries. Serve immediately.

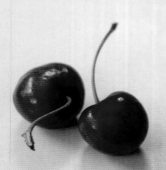

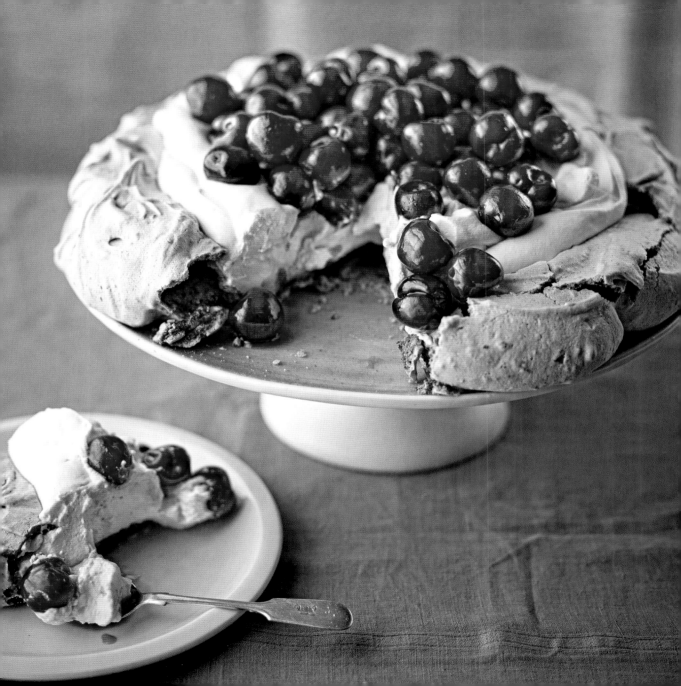

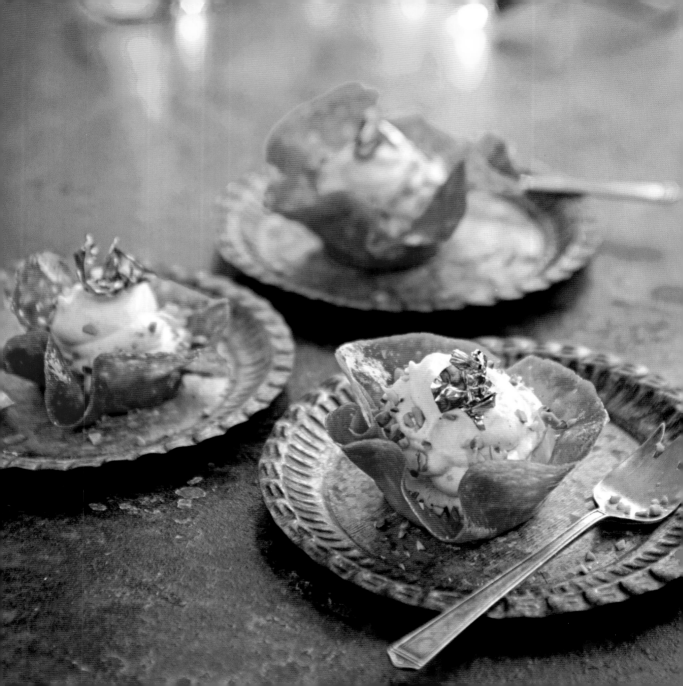

These snaps, a true 1970s throwback, are shaped into baskets and filled with a Christmasy syllabub, scented with cinnamon, lemon and ginger, and topped with shimmering gold leaf.

brandy snap baskets with spiced syllabub

for the brandy snap baskets

60 g/4 tablespoons butter

60 g/4 tablespoons caster/superfine sugar

60 g/¼ cup golden syrup/light corn syrup

60 g/½ cup plain/all-purpose gluten-free flour, sifted

for the syllabub

120 ml/½ cup green ginger wine

grated zest and freshly squeezed juice of 1 lemon

80 g/⅓ cup caster/superfine sugar

1 teaspoon ground cinnamon

300 ml/1¼ cups double/heavy cream

1 egg white

to decorate

unsalted pistachios, finely chopped

edible gold leaf

a large baking sheet, lined with a silicone mat

4 glass tumblers, inverted and bases greased with butter

makes 8

Preheat the oven to 180°C (350°F) Gas 4.

For the brandy snap baskets, heat the butter, sugar and syrup in a saucepan over a gentle heat, until the butter has melted and the sugar has dissolved. Remove the saucepan from the heat, and stir in the flour. Using half the mixture, place four large spoonfuls a large distance apart on the prepared baking sheet, as they will spread during cooking.

Bake in the preheated oven for 10–12 minutes, until they turn a golden orange colour. Remove from the oven and allow to set for a few minutes on the baking sheet. They should be firm enough to move without stretching, but still flexible enough to shape. If they set too hard, simply return to the oven for a minute to soften.

Using a palette knife, lift each biscuit/cookie over the base of a prepared glass tumbler, and press down so that each biscuit/cookie takes the shape of the glass and makes a basket. Leave on the glasses until cool while you bake the remaining batter in the same way, then make a further four baskets. The baskets will store in an airtight container for up to 5 days.

For the syllabub, place the wine, lemon zest and juice, sugar and cinnamon in a bowl, and leave to soak for 1 hour, until the sugar dissolves, stirring occasionally. Place the sugar syrup in a mixing bowl with the double/heavy cream, and whisk together to stiff peaks.

Place the egg white in a separate clean bowl, and whisk to stiff peaks. Gently fold the egg white into the cream mixture. Divide the syllabub between the brandy snap baskets, sprinkle with pistachios and top with a little gold leaf. Serve immediately.

The base of this trifle is made with a gluten-free Swiss/jelly roll, swirled with raspberry jam, which looks very pretty.

proper sherry trifle

for the trifle sponge

5 eggs

140 g/²⁄₃ cup caster/superfine sugar, plus extra for sprinkling

a pinch of vanilla salt (or 1 teaspoon pure vanilla extract and a pinch of salt)

100 g/²⁄₃ cup self-raising/rising gluten-free flour

1 teaspoon gluten-free baking powder

60 g/²⁄₃ cup ground almonds

4 tablespoons raspberry jam/jelly

for the fruit

350 g/2½ cups blueberries

1 tablespoon caster/superfine sugar

300 g/2 cups fresh raspberries

to assemble

125 ml/½ cup brandy

125 ml/½ cup sherry

500 ml/2 cups ready-made cold custard

400 ml/1²⁄₃ cups double/heavy cream, whipped to soft peaks

pomegranate seeds

a Swiss/jelly roll pan lined with baking parchment

large glass serving bowl

serves 10

Preheat the oven to 180°C (350°F) Gas 4.

For the sponge, whisk together the eggs, caster/superfine sugar and vanilla salt in a large mixing bowl for 3–5 minutes, using an electric mixer, until thick, creamy and pale. Sift together the flour and baking powder in a separate bowl, add the ground almonds, and fold into the egg mixture using a spatula. Fold very gently, otherwise you will lose all the air whipped into the eggs, which gives the roll its light texture.

Spoon the mixture into the lined Swiss/jelly roll pan and bake in the preheated oven for 5 minutes, then turn the tin around and cook for a further 3–5 minutes, until the sponge is golden-brown and feels just firm to your touch. Sprinkle a generous amount of caster/superfine sugar onto a sheet of baking parchment. Turn the sponge out onto the sugar-dusted sheet, and cover with a clean, damp kitchen cloth. Leave for 5 minutes. Remove the kitchen cloth and carefully peel off the bottom baking parchment (which is now on top). Mix the jam/jelly with a spoon, so that it is easily spreadable, then spread it over the sponge. Roll up the sponge from one of the long ends (as you want to make small swirls of sponge), using the sugar-dusted parchment to guide the sponge. Leave the Swiss/jelly roll wrapped in the parchment, until cool.

For the fruit, simmer half the blueberries in a saucepan with 60 ml/ ¼ cups water and the caster/superfine sugar for 5 minutes, until the fruit is soft and the liquid is syrupy. Allow to cool.

To assemble your trifle, cut the roll into slices and press into the base and sides of your glass bowl. Drizzle over the brandy and sherry – adding more if you like. Spoon the blueberry compote onto the base of the trifle, then sprinkle over the remaining blueberries and the raspberries. Spoon over the custard, then top with a layer of whipped cream. Sprinkle with the pomegranate seeds. Chill for at least 3 hours before serving. The trifle will keep for 3 days, covered, in the refrigerator.

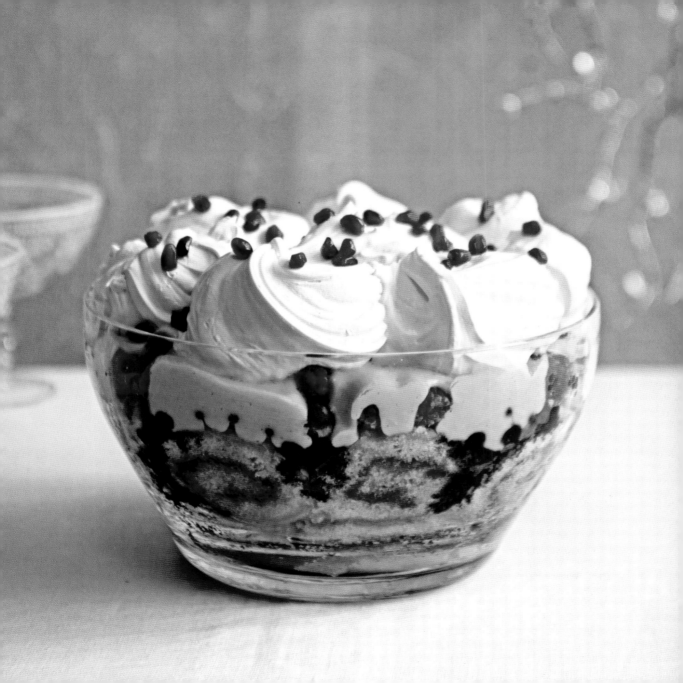

index

recipe credits

Miranda Ballard
Chicken breast wrapped in prosciutto with griddled chicory
Chilli con carne
Chorizo & scallop skewers
Cornichons wrapped in salami
Mozzarella pearls wrapped in salami
Perfectly tender pork chops
Pork & apple sliders
Pork stroganoff
Shepherd's pie
Sliced coppa and spring onion frittata
Sushi style prosciutto wrapped goats' cheese & rocket

Jordan Bourke
Coconut rice pudding with blueberries & maple syrup
Cod fish fingers with mushy peas & mayonnaise
Chocolate & pistachio cake with salted caramel
Farinata with red pepper & tender-stem broccoli
Halibut and coconut creamed corn with pak choi & chilli oil
Sea bass, cauliflower pureé and Swiss chard
Spiced chicken with quinoa, lemon zest & rose petals

Jordan & Jessica Bourke
Aubergine & tomato gratin
Sweet potato, cavolo nero & plum tomato frittata with basil oil

Ursula Ferrigno
Bean, lemon & herb potato cakes
Harissa pork with lime, radish, carrot & mint salad
Lemon cardamom & raspberry torte
Mango & lime jellies
Monkfish and bay skewers with lemon & vegetable slaw
Roast chicken with broad beans & lemon
Roasted hake, white beans & padron peppers
Salmon & kaffir lime cakes

Salmon escabeche with celery & citrus
Seared beef salad
Tandoori lamb cutlets with tomato & coriander salsa

Amy Ruth Finegold
Buckwheat & flaxseed pancakes
Coconut chia pudding
Dairy-free blueberry heaven yogurt muffins
Pineapple bran muffins

Mat Follas
Anchovy & potato gratin
Asparagus risotto
Braised red cabbage & burnt aubergine baba ganoush
Haddock with potato cakes, poached egg & hollandaise sauce
Mackerel kedgeree
Potato bowls with mushroom, garlic, spinach & ricotta
Savoy cabbage ratatouille parcels
Teriyaki salmon
Waldorf salad wraps

Liz Franklin
Aubergine & tomato toothpicks
Candied pineapple & stem ginger florentines

Victoria Glass
Black forest pavlova

Dunja Gulin
Castagnaccio cake
Coffee granita with whipped coconut cream
Fresh broad bean falafel
Fruit yogurt brekkie
Gluten-free bread

Victoria Hall
Apple crumble
Brownies
Carrot cake
Cheese & rosemary scones
Classic scones
Coconut crème brulée
Elderflower jelly fizz
Key lime pie
Lemon poppy seed drizzle loaf
Lemon posset
Malt loaf
Parmesan & poppy seed crisps
Peach cobbler
Raspberry & redcurrant roulade

Rocky road
Salmon & pea quiche
Sausage rolls
Spiced lentil & spinach pasties
Steak & ale pie
Victoria sponge cake

Carole Hilker
Quinoa porridge with maple syrup & brown sugar

Jenny Linford
Baked mushroom & egg ramekins
Beauf borguignon
Chicken caccitore
Greek rice-stuffed tomatoes
Griddled tuna with garlic bean purée & gremolata
Meatballs in spiced tomato sauce
Mushroom & bean chilli
Mushroom & halloumi kebabs
Polenta puttanesca
Polenta with wild mushrooms
Puy lentils in sage & tomato sauce
Saffron garlic chicken kebabs
Tofu & mushroom hotpot
Tricolore mushroom frittata
Tunisian baked eggs in tomato sauce
Yakitori-glazed mushrooms & chicken skewers

Hannah Miles
Introduction
Beef wellington
Blue cheese & walnut dip with celery
Brandy snap baskets with spiced syllabub
Cheese & bacon bread pudding
Cheese & onion soufflé muffins
Chorizo & manchego scones
Courgette bread
English muffins with eggs benedict
French onion dip with homemade potato crisps
Olive oil crackers
Proper sherry trifle
Smoked haddock scotch eggs
Steak & kidney pudding
Taleggio & hazelnut loaf cakes
Thyme flower mushrooms
Toad in the hole

Rosa Rigby
Frangipane tray bake
Lemon thyme & pink peppercorn steak

Mocha mousse
Pesto pasta

Laura Washburn
Aubergine & sumac fries

Jenna Zoe
Power protein granola

picture credits

Peter Cassidy
p10, 30, 100, 112, 115, 123, 124, 150, 216

Laura Edwards
p223

Tara Fisher
p85, 86, 111, 148, 165, 225, 226

Dan Jones
p204, 233

Mowie Kay
p46, 49, 50, 61, 139, 157, 188, 189, 229

Adrian Lawrence
p34, 65, 66, 70, 120, 172-182, 186, 193, 197, 206-210, 213, 214, 217, 221

Steve Painter
p2, 32, 38, 42, 45, 53, 54, 58, 69, 74, 89, 97, 98, 102, 104, 108, 128, 132, 135, 136, 153-155, 161

William Reavell
p5, 8, 22, 26, 36, 37, 41, 62, 63, 79, 91, 95, 102, 103, 140-147, 194, 198, 201, 202, 205, 227, 228, 230, 234, 237

Kate Whitaker
p1, 13, 28, 29, 31, 39, 83, 118, 119, 133, 158, 184, 190, 195, 203, 211, 232

Clare Winfield
p3, 4, 9, 14, 17-21, 25, 33, 57, 60, 68, 72, 73, 77, 78, 80-82, 90, 93, 94, 101, 107, 116, 117, 127, 130, 131, 149, 151, 162, 163, 166-171, 185, 218, 219, 222